What's Wrong With My Dog or Puppy?

John Rossi DVM MA

The What's Wrong Library®

1st Edition
Published by: What's Wrong Publishing Company
2641 Park Street
Jacksonville, Florida USA 32204

All Photographs by the author.

Printed in the United States of America

ISBN 978-0-9818072-8
Distributed in the United States by:
What's Wrong Publishing Company
Fax: (904) 388-2280 Web Site: Whatswrongwithmy.net

Dedication

This book is dedicated to my parents, Dr. Roscoe and Rosalind Rossi. Not only did they tolerate all of my childhood animal related adventures, but they encouraged them. Thanks Mom and Dad!

Acknowledgements

I would like to thank all of my staff who put up with my extra-curricular activities, including putting this book and others together, while working for me. I would also like to thank my clients who tolerated me being late, tired or even absent on occasions, while I was engaged in these activities. Well everyone, here are some of the results of those times. It wouldn't or couldn't have happened without your patience. Thank you so much. I promise I'll be there right after I take care of that next emergency.

I want to thank all of my teachers and colleagues who shared their knowledge with me and demonstrated their patience and persistence. You are a cut above and I have the greatest respect for you.

Dr. Alan Weldon DVM, DACVIM, reviewed the manuscript and made many helpful suggestions

Sofi Moss and John C. Rossi, copy edited the manuscript.

Roxanne Henkle diligently made many corrections necessary to complete this book.

What's Wrong with My Dog?

TABLE OF CONTENTS

What's Wrong With My Dog?

John Rossi DVM MA

Introduction

The dog *Canis familiaris* , is the most popular pet in the world. If your family pet had a problem, would you know how to recognize it and help your trusted friend until you could get professional help? Maybe it is a problem you could solve yourself! This book will help. There are many different problems and it will be difficult to discuss every contingency. In fact, to make this book more effective, I have left out comprehensive discussions of each problem and focused on the most likely causes for each problem. Nevertheless, this book will discuss the major problems. The same approach that has been used in other books in this series has been utilized here. That is, the common name of the problems are discussed in alphabetical order i.e. constipation, diarrhea, etc. This results in a rapid access recognition approach which may save lives. Quick and common sense solutions to these problems are discussed and the reader is advised when professional help is required. The book is also well illustrated, which helps in recognition of the problems discussed. As with all books in the series, it is inexpensive, concise, and life saving. Where certain events are known to have occurred (i.e. drowning, insect bites, smoke inhalation, etc...), the first aid treatment is covered in some detail.

For dog owners, it will be an essential addition to their library. This book is not an inclusive treatise on all of the diseases and treatments of dogs. Rather it is a brief summary of the most common signs, their likely meaning, and first aid for these problems.

There is also a section on preventive maintenance and a chart of drugs commonly used in dogs. In addition, there is a list of items suggested for a dog first aid kit and a Problem/Solution chart. A number of references on dogs and helpful websites are listed as well. Again this is not an inclusive list of references and websites. The phone numbers of several veterinary poison control centers are listed following these helpful websites.

Abdominal Swelling

The major reasons for abdominal swelling include heart disease, liver disease or abdominal fat. Other causes include parasitism, particularly in puppies, or adrenal disease in older dogs. Of course, don't forget the possibility of pregnancy in a young unspayed female! Lastly, the sudden onset of abdominal swelling may be a very serious problem called bloat. With the exception of treating a young dog for worms, or making a pregnant dog comfortable during delivery, none of these problems are easily diagnosed or treated at home, so get that dog to a veterinarian right away. This is especially true if there are any other signs accompanying the abdominal swelling. Signs such as coughing or exercise intolerance along with abdominal swelling suggest that a dog may be in congestive heart failure. Jaundice, a yellow discoloration of the skin and mucous membranes is a strong indicator of liver disease. In combination with abdominal swelling, jaundice may be even more serious, and a liver tumor is possible. Lethargy may accompany both of these problems. Conversely, if a dog is not lethargic and has shown a gradual increase in abdominal girth along with a significant appetite and limited exercise, fat is the prime suspect. Of course, this is not an emergency but needs to be addressed at some point. **Fig. 1, Fig. 2, Fig. 3**

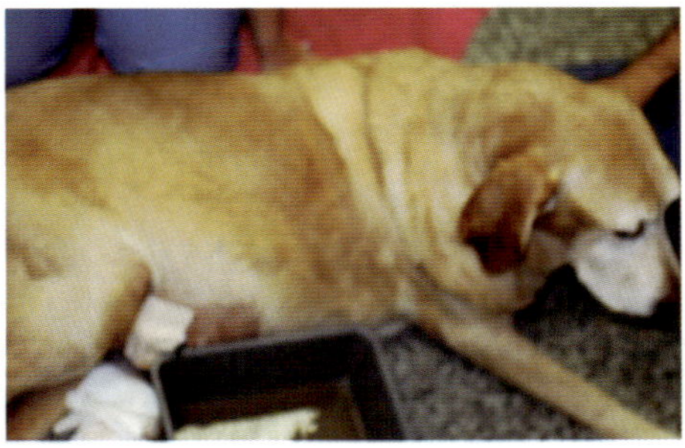

Fig. 1. Abdominal swelling due to ascites (fluid in the abdomen). In this case it was due to congestive heart failure.

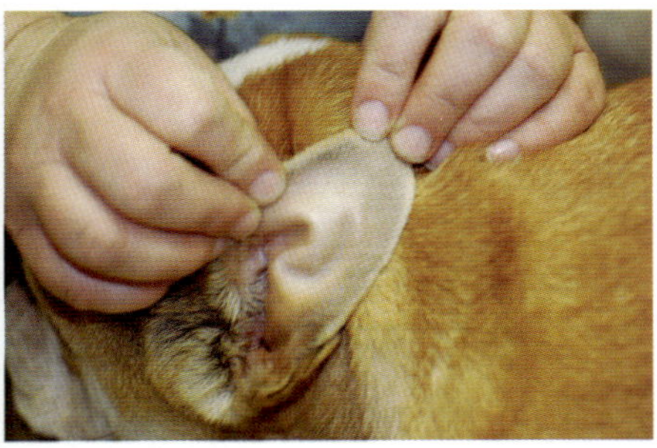

Fig. 2. Jaundice a yellow discoloration of the skin and mucous membranes associated with liver disease.

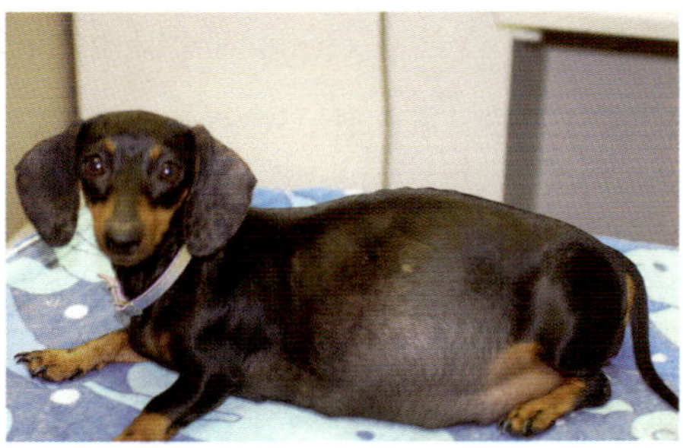

Fig. 3. Abdominal swelling associated with pregnancy.

Bloat requires a separate discussion. Rapid swelling of the abdomen may be due to a situation in which the stomach twists and traps gas produced by bacteria. The swelling and twisting results in a circulatory system emergency referred to as shock. You may confirm your suspicions by gently tapping the abdomen behind the last ribs. If it sounds hollow like a drum, this problem is likely. Also, you may observe the dog repeatedly attempt to vomit, but without success. **You must get that dog to a veterinarian immediately. Stomach decompression and possibly surgery may be required. If you can't get the dog to a veterinarian right away, you may try to pass a stomach tube yourself.[1] Place something in the mouth to keep the dog from biting down and pass the tube behind the canine teeth If the tube gets into the stomach, air will be forcefully expelled. If coughing occurs, pull out the tube and try again.**

Adrenal disease is fairly rare compared to the other problems listed above, but if there are significant skin problems, it may be suspected. Again, this is not a problem that can be diagnosed and treated at home. **Get your pet to the vet right away.**

To summarize, the majority of the reasons for abdominal swelling are not easily diagnosed or treated at home. Get the family veterinarian involved right away.

Anorexia

There are a very large number of reasons that a dog may refuse to eat. Everything from emotional distress due to the loss of a family member (animal or human) to the most serious of medical conditions is possible. Bacterial or viral diseases, intestinal blockage, tumors, parasites, metabolic diseases or exposure to a toxin are all possible causes, among others. Acute anorexia, which is defined as that lasting less than 24 hours, is a very common problem and generally not a big concern unless you are dealing with a very small dog or the dog is showing other signs of illness such as vomiting, diarrhea, coughing, etc... Offer a small treat, and if it is consumed, it is usually a self limiting problem. If not, the problem may progress to chronic anorexia, which can be the harbinger of a serious problem, as listed above.

In my experience, the most common cause for anorexia is what we call acute dietary indiscretion, or to translate... the dog ate something he or she shouldn't have! Thus, there may be either a bacterial toxemia (food poisoning) or a physical impediment (a partial or total blockage) or both. Vomiting or

1. Stomach tubes maybe purchased from the veterinarians in advance.

diarrhea may accompany either of these problems, but not necessarily. Generally speaking, if the patient is not depressed or lethargic, one may attempt to manage this problem conservatively for a few days. This would include the administration of a bulk laxative like Metamucil® two to three times a day along with a GI protectant like kaolin/pectin (Kaopectate®). The doses are listed in the drug chart. **If no appetite returns after one to two days, it is time to seek professional help.** There may be a serious problem. A veterinarian may run bloodwork or take a radiograph (X-ray) in order to determine the cause. One of the first signs of the deadly parvo virus is a loss of appetite. This is soon followed by lethargy, fever, vomiting and diarrhea. Intestinal worms such as hookworms or roundworms may cause these signs as well.

Bad Breath

The number one reason for bad breath (halitosis) is dental disease. Tartar and infection of the gums, called gingivitis is likely. Lift up one of your dogs lips and look at the back teeth. If you see a buildup of material on any teeth, there is a problem. This is called tartar, which is a build up of minerals, food and bacteria. While some people may be able to brush their dog's teeth (and you should try with special dog toothpaste), it is necessary that they be cleaned professionally. This will usually require general anesthesia. Your veterinarian will scale the teeth, polish them and apply fluoride. **Fig. 4**

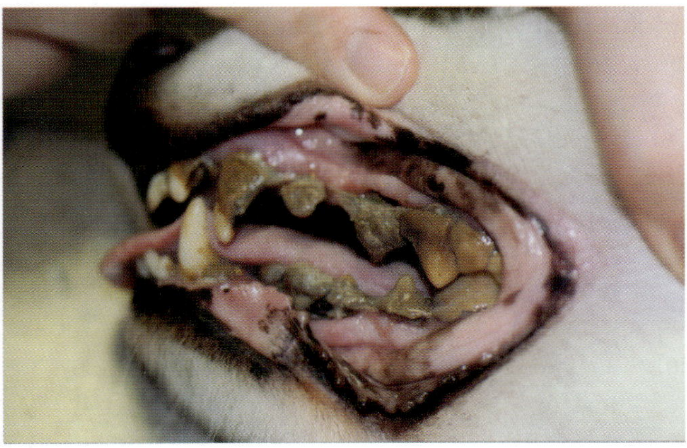

Fig. 4. Severe dental tartar and gingivitis may contribute to many health problems including heart disease.

Other causes for bad breath include metabolic problems such as liver or kidney disease or gastrointestinal problems, such as poor digestion or slow passage of food. These problems can only be diagnosed by a veterinarian, who will run bloodwork in order to determine if any organs are not functioning properly.

Chronic untreated dental disease may lead to severe inflammation of the gums and a pre-cancerous growth called epulis. These are cauliflower like structures that often bleed. They will aggravate the situation by trapping material and contributing to pain and discomfort, as well as odor. Certainly, any untreated dental disease may contribute to a painful situation, and this may be accompanied by excessive drooling.

Certain kinds of food may not agree with your dog i.e. Perhaps one of the ingredients is either hard for your dog to digest or actually initiates an allergic or irritating response. If this is the case, simply changing the food may solve the problem.

Behavioral Changes

Changes in behavior may be subtle or dramatic. In dogs, most behavioral changes are associated with a medical problem, but they are not specific i.e. A change in behavior may be associated with a variety of medical problems. These may include everything from a stomach ache to a brain tumor. Examples of medical problems leading to behavioral changes are metabolic problems, such as diabetes or hypothyroidism, liver or kidney disease, as well as toxicity, parasitism, cancer, infection, or trauma. Even dental disease can result in a change in behavior. Indeed, a dog that is in pain or discomfort is more likely to become irritable and perhaps bite if it is touched.

Strictly psychological problems are less common causes of behavioral changes than medical problems, but they do occur. Even a single frightening event may change a dog's behavior in an unexpected way. Examples abound, such as fireworks on the Fourth of July or scarily dressed children on Halloween, causing a fearful response in some animals. The addition of a new animal to the household, or the loss of an owner or longtime animal friend are also very likely to result in a major change in behavior. In addition, the behavior of older dogs may change. Typically, older dogs may become less active; their senses less acute, and their patience with changing people or routines much lower. Sound familiar? Extremes of behavior change in older dogs (e.g. disorientation, lack of response, wandering) may suggest a problem called cognitive dysfunction syndrome. This is a medical problem and there is a medication that may help called selegiline (Anipryl®).

One of the recently recognized syndromes that appears to be a common behavioral problem is separation anxiety. An affected dog may become extremely destructive or bark incessantly when you leave your home. Treatment may require a program of conditioning your dog not to be fearful or upset when you have to leave the home. This may involve a series of fun things to do whenever you have to leave. Turn on the radio, give some sort of a positive distraction, pretend you are leaving and then come right back. Then do it for longer and longer periods. Positive distractions may include a Kong® toy stuffed with some peanut butter or some other treat. A Greenie® may work well for this purpose. A steak bone with a little meat left on it will distract even the most fearful dog! Sometimes however, medications such as tricyclic antidepressants like clomipramine (Clomicalm®) or amitryptiline (Elavil®) or SSRIs like fluoxetine (Prozac®) or paroxetine (Paxil®) will be needed along with a conditioning program. Other dogs may respond to another class of drugs such as the benzodiazepines, which include diazepam (Valium®) or clonazepam (Klonopin®). The doses for all of these drugs are listed in the drug chart.

Natural products which have been shown to have some calming influence include St. John's Wort, melatonin, and SAM-e. The plug-in that produces dog pheromones, called DAP®, has helped calm dogs down fairly well in some cases.

Sometimes, people unintentionally encourage the behavior they are trying to prevent. When you comfort a dog during a storm, you reinforce their fears about storms. Ignore the storm. Act happy and relaxed and offer a very positive distraction...small amounts of a favored food for instance. If the food is a real treat, it won't be long before your dog looks forward to storms! You can also desensitize a dog to storms and other loud noises by playing a CD of a storm at a very low volume level and gradually (over days or weeks) turning it up.

In any case, any change in behavior should be viewed as a potentially serious problem, and one should seek veterinary help and possibly a dog trainer immediately.

Bites (and Abscesses)

Dogs fight. Bite wounds may be inflicted and some of these bite wounds may become infected. If the wound remains closed, an abscess may form. An abscess is basically a pus filled pocket. In order to heal, this pus must drain. This may either occur naturally in some cases, or need help to drain in many cases. In some cases the tissue around the abscess may become very swollen. This is called cellulitis and it is a very frightening thing for the owner to witness in their pet. Sometimes a leg may become swollen to twice its normal size. **Fig. 5**

Therefore, all bites should be treated as infected wounds, with abscesses either present or likely to occur soon. The best way to deal with these wounds is to apply warm compresses to them twice daily for 5 to 10 minutes each time. Antibiotics may be required in order to eliminate this infection, and amoxi-

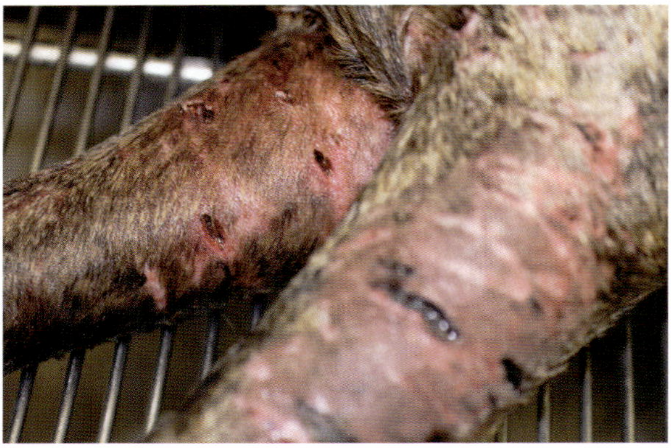

Fig. 5. Bite wounds can become very swollen and infected and much of the damage may be concealed.

cillin or cephalexin usually are very effective. **Warning: A small puncture wound on the surface may be accompanied by a huge amount of trauma beneath it, including torn muscles, severe bruising, damaged organs or internal bleeding! If there are any doubts, seek professional help immediately. Veterinarians refer to this as the "iceberg effect". This is especially important when a small dog has been attacked by a big dog. Keep in mind that a veterinarian may recommend exploring the wound surgically to repair the damage done. Follow their recommendations.**

First aid for recent bites would include cleaning the wounds, making sure there is no active bleeding, and reducing the pain by administering an analgesic like Rimadyl®, Metacam® or aspirin at the doses listed in the drug chart. Do not give aspirin if there is any evidence of continued bleeding. Applying ice may be helpful for about an hour. The application of heat may be useful after 24 hours.

Bleeding

Bleeding from any location is always an emergency. One should always attempt to stop bleeding by applying pressure to the site immediately with a soft absorbent material, such as gauze or a washcloth. In the absence of any material, just apply pressure. If the bleeding can't be stopped or if major blood loss has occurred, get your dog to a veterinarian right away. In the case of a torn and bleeding toenail, one may attempt to dip the bleeding nail into some sort of powder, such as flour or cornstarch, or even better, styptic powder. Bar soap also works well in some cases. Simply press the nail into the soap, and the bleeding will often be stopped. Cyanoacrylate glues (e.g. Superglue®), produced by many different manufacturers, have also been used to stop bleeding. These glues may burn however, so be prepared for a negative response from the dog. A small laceration may actually be pulled together and the bleeding stopped by using these glues in combination with some medical tape or even a Band-Aid®.

Once the bleeding has been stopped, a decision needs to be made as to whether the wound needs to be closed or can heal as an open wound. Generally speaking, small wounds (approximately 2.5 cm long by 1.25 cm wide or 1 inch long by ½ inch wide) may be left open and they will heal within several weeks if they are kept relatively clean. Wounds larger than that are probably best closed as soon as possible. Keep in mind that there is a time limit. Doctors refer to this time during which a wound can be closed as the "golden period", and it is about seven hours.

Internal bleeding is less obvious, but just as serious. In dogs, there are four major causes. These include: 1. Blunt trauma to the thorax or abdomen 2. A bleeding thoracic or abdominal tumor 3. An autoimmune disease 4. Rat poison or other anticoagulant poison consumption. The gums may suddenly turn pale and the dog may collapse.

Bleeding from the nose, mouth, ears, urinary openings or rectum is a very serious sign. It may suggest a variety of problems. These are all emergencies and they need to be addressed immediately by a veterinarian. Get that dog to a veterinarian right away! Keep the dog quiet and calm and transport immediately. Fig. 6

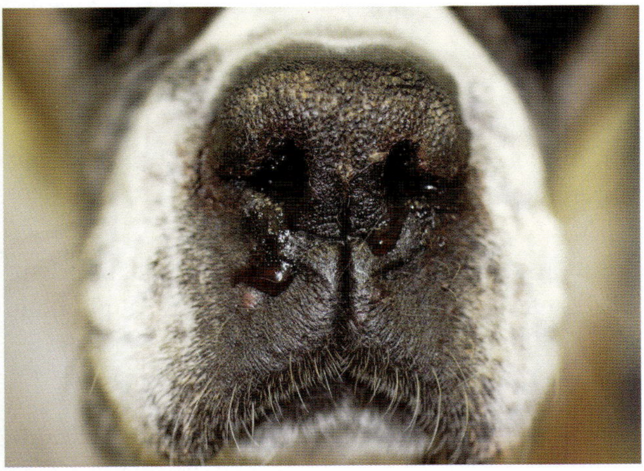

Fig. 6. Hemorrhage from the nose is very serious and could represent toxicity, blood parasitism or an autoimmune disease.

An unusual manifestation of internal bleeding is the presence of red or dark red spots under the skin. This may look like a group of bruises and they may be generalized (widespread around the whole body). These are referred to as petechial hemorrhages and they are a very serious sign which usually means that there is a clotting problem. There are a variety of reasons that this may occur and they all require professional help to diagnose and treat. **Fig. 7**

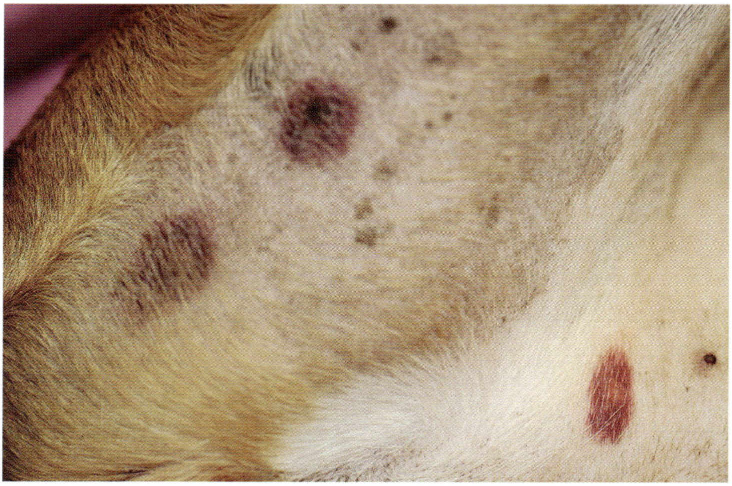

Fig. 7. Petechial hemorrhages or small bleeding areas under the skin may be caused by the same things that cause frank bleeding from the nose, mouth or rectum. This is a serious sign.

Breathing Problems (Dyspnea)

Regardless of the cause, rapid or difficult breathing is always a serious sign. In dogs, the majority of respiratory problems seen are infectious. Infectious tracheobronchitis, also known as kennel cough, is a very common reason for dogs to begin coughing. It is often associated with a fever and a discharge from the nose and eyes. Sometimes they struggle to breathe. See the section on coughing. Other infectious diseases are possible, including a variety of viruses and bacteria, as well as fungi. Bacterial pneumonia may occur, and this is a possible cause of difficult breathing.

Many breathing problems in dogs are associated with heart problems. Heart disease often leads to CHF (congestive heart failure), in which fluids build up in the chest or abdomen. This may also be caused by heartworms. Rapid breathing, coughing and exercise intolerance are the most common signs.

Other causes for difficult breathing include asthma, small airway disease (a genetic predisposition to have small airways, whether it be narrow nostrils or a narrow trachea (even in some cases, a collapsing trachea). Chronic bronchitis or pulmonary neoplasia (a lung tumor) are also possible causes for breathing difficulties. A foreign object lodged in the trachea may create a situation in which breathing becomes very difficult and is associated with coughing. Any history of foreign object consumption should be reported to your veterinarian.

Overheating or overeating may also cause rapid breathing. A large dog that suddenly develops rapid breathing right after eating a big meal may be experiencing gastric torsion (a twisted stomach). If the belly is tense and appears bloated, this should be suspected.

Every case of difficult breathing should be considered an emergency and the dog should be taken to a veterinarian, where the cause may be determined and treated as soon as possible. There is little that can be done at home to remedy the situation without knowing the cause, and this may require radiographs and bloodwork.

CPR

Cardiopulmonary resuscitation is a series of techniques that may be utilized to "jump start" the heart and lungs of a dog, whose heart and lungs have just ceased to function. The new term for this is CPCR, which stands for cardiopulmonary cerebral resuscitation. This term indicates the importance of maintaining cerebral circulation as well as that of the heart and lungs. In veterinary hospitals, this function might be helped by the rapid IV administration of large volumes of fluids, but not necessarily. From a practical first aid standpoint, this is not an option that is available. **Therefore, the first and most important thing one can do is to compress the chest rapidly. Recent recommendations suggest that 100 compressions per minute with a 1/1 compression to relaxation ratio is best (Hanel, 2008). Ideally, the dog should be placed on its right side. The next step would be to ventilate the dog (breathe for the dog). However, in the case of very large dogs, this may not be easy. Sometimes you may be able to place your hand around the closed mouth to form a "cone" with your thumb and forefinger around a large dog's nose. Pull the tongue as far forward as you can during the entire process. Then you may breathe into the cone you have formed. With small dogs this is relatively easy. If working by yourself, ventilations can be administered as often as every 5 chest compressions for a small dog or as infrequently as every thirty chest compressions for a large dog. If you have help, the person breathing should administer 10 to 12 breaths per minute (Hanel, 2008). Keep the neck straight during this process and look for the chest to inflate and deflate. If heartbeat and breathing resume, transport to a veterinarian right away. Keep in mind however, that less than 10% of CPCR attempts are successful.**

CPR Summary

1. **Place dog on right side.**
2. **Place one hand over the other and compress the widest part of the chest 80 – 100 times per minute with a 1/1 compression to relaxation ratio.**
3. **Form a cone with your hand to close the mouth and "frame" the nose.**
4. **Pull the tongue as far forward as you can.**
5. **Straighten out the neck.**
6. **Breathe forcefully into the nose after every 5 chest compressions (if working by yourself on a small dog or after every 30 compressions in a large dog).**
7. **Watch for the chest to inflate and deflate during and after the breathing attempt. If the chest does not inflate, try forming a tighter cone with your hand and breathe more forcefully into the nose.**

Collapse

When a dog collapses, it is frightening to observe regardless of the cause. Likely causes include heart disease, anemia, internal hemorrhage, shock, a seizure, low blood sugar (hypoglycemia), low blood calcium (hypocalcemia) and a variety of other things. This is not something that can be diagnosed or treated at home. Get your dog to a veterinarian right away! Keep your dog warm and make him or her as comfortable as possible, but seek professional help immediately. Give some sugar water to small dogs or puppies if they are capable of drinking, but do not hesitate to get all dogs that have collapsed to a veterinarian right away. In some cases an older dog may bang a friable (fragile) internal organ and be bleeding so rapidly inside they are difficult to save, even with professional help…so again, **do not hesitate. Get that dog to a veterinarian right away.**

Shaking often accompanies collapse. This does not change the situation from a diagnostic or treatment perspective. It must be diagnosed by a veterinarian. *See the section on shaking*. Perhaps one of the more easily recognized reasons for collapse and shaking however, is that seen with a nursing mother. If a bitch with a litter of puppies (particularly a small dog) collapses and begins shaking, she is probably suffering from a lack of calcium. Her muscles will often twitch uncontrollably and generate a lot of heat in the process. This is also known as "milk fever." Remove the puppies from the mother immediately and plan to bottle feed them for a while. Again, cover her and get her to a veterinarian right away. If no help is immediately available, give lactose free, low fat milk to a dog that is still capable of drinking. This is a good source of absorbable calcium. Keep in mind that this may only help in mild cases. **See a veterinarian!** They will administer a calcium supplement intravenously until the shaking stops. After recovery, give a calcium supplement like Pet Cal® or one of the human calcium supplements. Make sure that she is eating a good quality puppy food because most of these diets are high in calcium and protein, which will help her recover more quickly. In some cases, you may not be able to allow the puppies to continue nursing and they may have to be bottle fed until they are weaned. Begin offering them solid food (moistened in a milk replacer) as early as three weeks of age.

Constipation

If a dog has not defecated for more than two days, it may be constipated. Several approaches to this problem are available. All laxatives used by people are suitable for use in the dog. Furthermore the dose is the same as it is in people. Metamucil® crackers are particularly useful, since most dogs readily consume them. One to two crackers may be given every 4 hours until results are observed. Canned pumpkin has also proven to be very effective in achieving the same response. Several teaspoons given with each meal will often relieve the constipation. More serious cases may be managed with the help of a veterinarian. An enema may be required to solve this problem. For many dogs, this may require sedation. A stool softener like Colace® may also be required or helpful for long term prevention of constipation. The dose is listed in the drug chart.

Coughing

Coughing may be a serious sign in the dog. There are five basic causes for coughing in the dog. These are infectious (bacterial, viral, fungal), cardiogenic (heart related), allergic, structural (a collapsing trachea or elongated soft palate) and neoplastic (cancer).

A general rule is that coughing "fits" or multiple coughs suggest that there is a respiratory system problem while single coughs suggest a heart problem! Another observation is that a dog with a heart problem may breathe rapidly even while it is resting. A dog with a respiratory problem is usually breathing at a normal rate when it is resting.

As mentioned in the section on difficult breathing, coughing may be caused by an infectious agent. The most common bacterial cause for coughing is *Bordetella bronchiseptica*, the cause of kennel cough. This is a close relative of *Bordetella pertussis*, the cause of whooping cough in people. This cough is a harsh, hacking cough and it is often productive. That means that sputum is often ejected from the mouth. Many people confuse this with vomiting but food is rarely involved unless the coughing is so severe that a gag reflex is activated. This cough is often associated with a fever of around 103° F, a greenish discharge from the eyes and a moderate loss of appetite. This contrasts sharply with a canine distemper infection, which is also a potential infectious cause of coughing. In the case of distemper, one may expect a fever of 105°F, a total loss of appetite, seizures, extreme discharge from the nose and usually death. Initially however, the two look similar.

First aid for a cough usually involves the use of a cough suppressant/expectorant. Any over the counter product that is marked for use in children can be used in dogs. Robitussin® has worked very well at the dose listed in the drug chart at the frequency recommended for children. Antibiotics may be very helpful for treating *Bordetella* infections or limiting their severity so see your veterinarian right away. Very little is successful in treating canine distemper. That is why vaccinations are so important.

Cardiogenic (heart related) causes for coughing are common in the dog. Basically, congestive heart failure results in a backup of blood into the blood vessels leading into the heart (either or both sides) and pressure building up in those blood vessels. If the backup occurs on the left side, pressure builds up in the lungs and the fluid exuded from the blood vessels causes pulmonary edema (fluid in the lungs). If the backup occurs on the right side, pressure builds up in the vena cava, liver, kidneys and the resultant fluid exuded ends up outside the lungs if deposited in the chest (called pleural effusion) or in the abdominal cavity (called ascites). The causes are numerous but involve either a failure of the valves of the heart or the muscles of the heart. Heartworms may also be responsible. In any case, this is not a problem that can be diagnosed by a layman. Thus, a veterinarian needs to be consulted. First aid invovles using diuretic agents (i.e. drugs that increase urination and eliminate excess fluids in the body). Almost all diuretic agents are prescription drugs, but there are a few things that may be helpful that are over the counter (OTC). These include coffee and tea, as well as a product named Disal®. But in my experience, congestive heart failure (CHF) requires immediate medical attention. Get your dog to a veterinarian right away.

Allergic bronchitis is a common source of coughing. Allergens may cause bronchoconstriction with resultant wheezing and coughing. There is no easy way to diagnose this. Observing these signs right after the exposure to a new habitat or substance would make one suspicious of this problem. If the body temperature is normal (101.5 – 102.5 ° F) and there is a clear discharge from the eyes rather than a yellow or green discharge, it is highly likely. An antihistamine such as diphenhydramine HCL at a dose of 2 mg/kg may be helpful, but one should seek professional help as soon as possible.

A structural (morphological) defect may contribute to a severe cough. The most obvious physical defect is a collapsing trachea, but this and other physical problems are impossible to diagnose without radiographs or endoscopy. This occurs much more commonly in small breed dogs. The cough is often described as a honking cough.

Dehydration

Chronic vomiting or diarrhea or a combination may result in a state of dehydration. Kidney disease may also be a cause of dehydration. Dehydration may be recognized by a reduction in skin turgor. That means that when the skin is pulled away from the body, it returns to its position very slowly. Veterinarians call this poor skin turgor. In combination with a dry mouth, it suggests that a dog is at least 5% dehydrated. More severe dehydration may be recognized by dry, red gums, weak pulse, and a reduction of urination. Obviously severe dehydration is a life threatening emergency. Get that dog to a veterinarian right away.

In cases of mild dehydration, the fluid required may be calculated fairly easily. If a dog is 5% dehydrated, multiply .05 times the dog's weight in kilograms. To get the weight in kg, divide the weight in pounds by 2.2. So a 44 pound dog, would be a 20 kg dog. Thus, 20 times .05 would equal 1 kg. This is equal to 1000 ml (1Liter) or approximately one quart (987 ml). If a dog is drinking and capable of keeping fluids without vomiting, this is what would be required to replace what is lost. If not, fluids will need to be replaced via IV(intravenous) or SQ (subcutaneous) fluid therapy. If the fluid loss is chronic, one also needs to consider the daily fluid requirements as well as the amount needed to replace the deficit mentioned above. For the average sized dog, the daily requirement is approximately 70 ml per kg per day, or 30 ml per pound per day. For smaller dogs, it is actually twice as much per kg; for very large dogs, it is one half as much per kg. So, a 1 kg dog (two pounds) would require 140 ml per day for maintenance, while a 100 kg dog (approximately 200 pounds) would require about 40 ml/kg or 4000 ml/day (4 liters) for maintenance. This is roughly one gallon.

To summarize, a twenty kg dog (44 pounds) that was 5% dehydrated would require one liter for the dehydration plus about 1400 ml per day for maintenance (20 kg times 70 ml/kg). Thus, on the first day, it might need as much as 2.4 liters, and each day afterwards, it would require 1.4 liters.

Obviously, water is the fluid of choice for mildly dehydrated animals that can keep it down. However, Pedialyte® and Gatorade® are excellent electrolyte supplementing fluids. A homemade rehydrating solution may be made by mixing 1 tablespoon of sugar and 1 teaspoon of salt into 1 liter (one quart) of water.

Keep in mind that the underlying cause of the dehydration must be determined by a veterinarian. They will run several tests to determine the cause and recommend a treatment for that underlying disease process.

Dental Disease

There are three main signs of dental disease in the dog. These are discoloration of the teeth, dental tartar and gingivitis.

Discoloration of the teeth may be internal or external. Internal staining suggests endodontal disease. One may think of this as a hematoma or a bruise that has occurred inside of a tooth. It may be due to trauma or infection. Antibiotics may be indicated if infection is suspected. In many cases, even if the infection is controlled or the trauma is over, the inside of the tooth remains stained.

Tartar, of course, is a deposit of minerals and bacteria on the tooth surface. Gingivitis is defined as inflammation of the gingival or gum line. Any inflammation around the teeth suggests that an infection is present and that it is painful for the dog. Reduced appetite is a common manifestation of dental disease. Occasionally a dog with dental disease will paw at its mouth, but this is not a consistent sign. Perhaps the most common and readily observable sign of gingivitis (also known as periodontal disease) is bad breath (halitosis), even though there are other causes for bad breath. **Fig. 8**

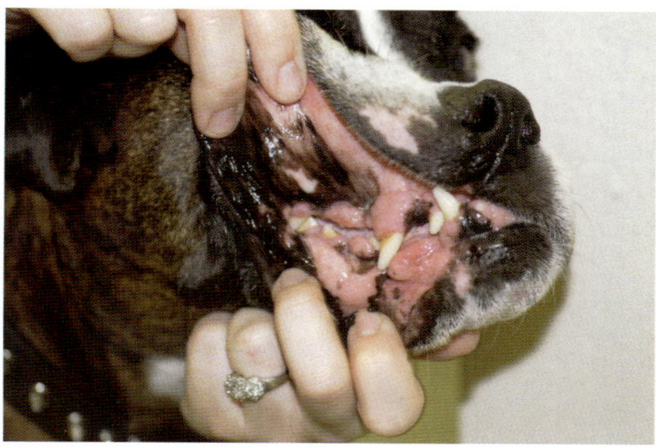

Fig. 8. Gingivitis and tartar with epulis (inflamed gum tissue).

First aid for dental disease involves reducing the dog's pain by using a topical oral pain medication as you would for a person with oral pain. A veterinarian will administer antibiotics and pain medications, and may suggest that a dental cleaning be performed under anesthesia. If a dog is very old, a veterinarian may choose to avoid anesthesia and treat the oral infection with antibiotics and pain meds only. Sometimes, however, infected teeth may need to be removed and this will require anesthesia.

Another kind of dental emergency is a chipped or fractured tooth. If a small chip is missing and the root canal is not exposed, no treatment is required. However, if the root canal is exposed, one may wish to consult a veterinarian who performs dentistry as soon as possible in an effort to save the tooth. Three outcomes appear possible: 1. A damaged infected tooth might need to be removed. 2. A root canal procedure may be performed to save the tooth. 3. Some teeth appear to autoseal. These teeth do not seem to become infected or painful! First aid for a fractured tooth until the dog can be seen would include pain medications such as aspirin, Rimadyl® or Metacam® at the doses in the drug chart.

Diarrhea

Loose stools are a common and potentially serious problem. Causes for diarrhea are numerous. These include everything from dietary indiscretion to abdominal cancer.

As mentioned in the section on anorexia, the ingestion of objects that "shouldn't be eaten" is common in dogs. The fancy name for this is "acute dietary indiscretion". This is also the most common reason for diarrhea and vomiting. If this is the case, the diarrhea of sudden onset, which is called acute diarrhea, may be managed somewhat conservatively. This means that we stop feeding anything for 12 to 24 hours, in order to allow the gut to "rest". Gastrointestinal protectants such as Kaopectate®, or Peptobismol® given at the doses listed in the drug chart are very helpful. Immodium® (loperamide) is also very successful at treating acute diarrhea. Refer to the drug chart for the dose. Once feeding is resumed, a bland diet should be offered first, and in small quantities. A bland food would be something like baked white meat chicken and rice, bread, baked potato, or plain pasta (cooked). Prescription Diet® I/D is also ideal for this purpose. A tablespoon of the food may be offered initially. If no vomiting or diarrhea occurs within an hour, offer another tablespoon, and so on for several small meals. If the diarrhea persists, stop feeding and seek professional help, and see below.

Another reason for acute (or chronic) diarrhea in dogs is intestinal parasitism.

The most common parasites are worms, which include hookworms, roundworms, whipworms, and tapeworms. Protozoal (one celled) parasites are also common and these include giardia, amoeba, and coccidia, among others. Worms may occasionally be recognized in the stool of an infected dog, but this is not reliable. A microscopic exam of the feces is often the only way to determine the presence of these parasites. See the section below on the worms and their treatment. Protozoans are never visible to the naked eye, and therefore the only way to diagnose them is via a microscopic examination of the feces by a veterinarian or veterinary technician. The treatment for these parasites depends upon the kind of parasites present. Therefore, any case of diarrhea lasting longer than 24 hours and non-responsive to conservative symptomatic therapy should be examined by a veterinarian.

More chronic cases of diarrhea are more difficult to diagnose and treat than acute cases. Causes of chronic diarrhea include a variety of diseases that cause either a failure to digest food (maldigestion), or a failure to absorb it (malabsorption). These may include inflammatory, infectious or neoplastic (cancer) causes. Since none of these can be diagnosed at home, all cases of chronic diarrhea require immediate veterinary attention to diagnose and treat. In the meantime, however, one may utilize the symptomatic treatment listed above in order to temporarily relieve the signs. A dietary change is sometimes required, either temporarily or permanently.

Dizziness

If a dog appears "drunk", there are a number of possible reasons. Veterinarians refer to this problem as ataxia. The major causes for ataxia are toxicity, anemia, hypoglycemia (low blood sugar), severe dehydration, a neurological deficit, or a cardiac problem. Recent trauma to the head may also cause this sign. **This problem cannot be diagnosed or treated at home. Get that dog to a veterinarian right away. That dog may be in imminent danger. The only first aid that can be administered at home is to rinse out the mouth repeatedly with a garden hose if the dog is known to have mouthed a toad or some other toxic substance.**

Occasionally, this is related to the ingestion of the owner's marijuana or other drug. Most veterinarians will not make any moral or legal judgments regarding the treatment of these animals. Be honest. Inform them of the possible ingestion, and allow them to provide supportive care. *See the discussion on Staggering.*

Dragging a Leg, Carrying a Leg, Limping

The loss of function of one leg may be caused by a fracture, nerve damage, muscle injury, or ligamentous injury.

The **sudden partial** loss of function is the most common kind of lameness. Generally speaking with this kind of injury, a dog is limping or "favoring" a leg(placing it down, but gingerly), but there are no obvious wounds or fractures. This is most likely a soft tissue injury, not a bone injury, and these are often manageable at home with non-steroidal anti-inflammatory drugs (NSAIDS) like buffered aspirin, Metacam®, or Rimadyl®, and rest. The doses are in the drug chart. If the lameness persists in spite of several days of this conservative approach, it is time to see the vet. **Fig. 9**

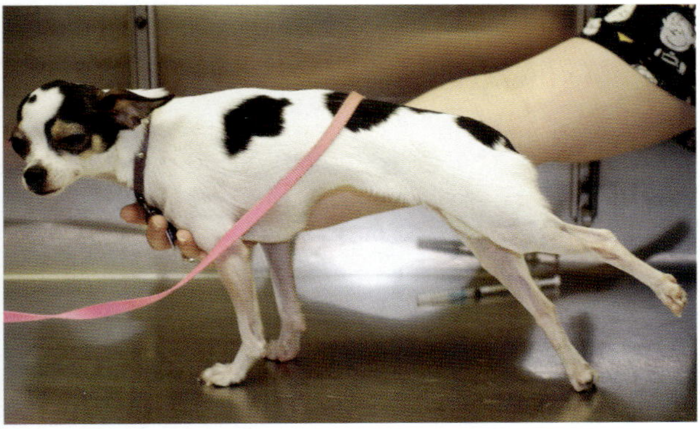

Fig. 9. Carrying a leg in this manner suggests a patellar luxation i.e. the kneecap is popping out of its normal location and "locking" towards one side or the other. Surgery will be required.

The **sudden complete** loss of function is more serious. Carrying a leg or dragging a leg suggests that there has been a fracture or nerve damage, or both. Carrying a leg may also occur with a dislocation. These problems should be diagnosed and treated by a veterinarian, although one may comfort a dog by administering one of the drugs listed above in order to help alleviate the pain until it can be seen. **Fig. 10**

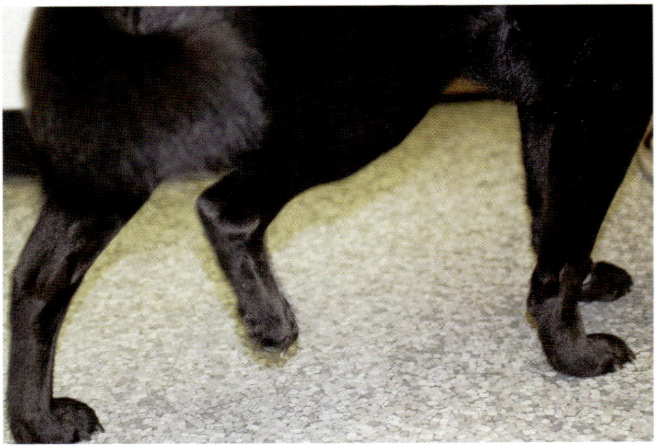

Fig. 10. The sudden onset of carrying a leg in this manner, and placing it down at times, suggests a sudden sprain or tear of the ACL (anterior cruciate ligament).

The dragging of a leg has its own ominous implications. It usually suggests that there has been some nerve damage. A dog may not be able to feel its own foot, and in some cases may appear to be walking on its knuckles. Veterinarians refer to this as "knuckling over". This may be temporary or permanent, but the foot will need to be protected from the damage done by dragging until the dog can be evaluated by a veterinarian. You may want to wrap the affected foot in a light bandage that will protect it from abrasion as it is dragged. The sooner these dogs are examined, the better their chances of being helped.

A gradual loss of function also has serious implications. While it may be something as common as arthritis, it may also represent the onset of a bone cancer or a bone infection. While temporary relief may be achieved by administering the anti-inflammatory drugs listed above, a veterinarian needs to be consulted as soon as possible.

Dragging the Rear Legs

The sudden dragging of the rear legs is a serious sign. In all dogs it suggests that there is some pressure on the spinal cord in the back. It may be traumatic, as in being hit by a car, or it may be degenerative, as in the case of degenerative disc disease, but it needs to be addressed immediately. In fact, if a dog suddenly starts dragging its rear legs and feels no pain in those legs, it is an emergency in which immediate surgical intervention will be necessary if the function of the legs is to be restored. This is usually seen in the case of "long backed" dogs like Dachshunds or Basset Hounds, and it is probably a ruptured intervertebral disc. These natural "shock absorbers" between the bones of the spine sometimes rupture, and the central part of the disc puts pressure on the spinal cord. If the pressure is great enough that it compresses even the central part of the spinal cord, then the dog feels absolutely no pain in its feet or legs. These dogs must be operated on within 24 – 48 hours or the loss of function may be permanent. However, if a dog is capable of walking, even weakly on its rear legs, or if it feels pain in its legs, it may be managed medically. One may determine if there is no pain by pinching a toe on the affected leg. If there is no response, get that dog to a veterinary surgeon right away.

The gradual onset of rear limb weakness is not an emergency, but it may suggest a degenerative process that may be treated by anti-inflammatory agents or other medicines and supplements. One of the less common degenerative problems leading to progressive weakness in the rear legs is called degenerative myelopathy. It is a degeneration of the myelin sheath that surrounds the spinal cord, and therefore interferes with its function. The problem is seen primarily in German Shepherds.

Ear Problems

Of all of the common problems that I deal with as a veterinarian, this group of problems is the most frustrating and most difficult I deal with. So many dogs suffer more from ear problems than all other problems combined. Ear problems are frequently ignored by owners and the dogs affected may suffer needlessly. Ear problems may be recognized either by observing certain behaviors or by noticing a discoloration of the area in or near the ears. Also a strong odor is often present when there is an ear infection. Aside from discolorations or discharges, you can observe swelling of the ear, redness, hair loss, lacerations, rashes and many other things.

Behaviors observed when ear problems are present include pawing or scratching at the ears, shaking the head, and sometimes a head tilt. A head tilt is usually to the side that is infected (or infected worse if both ears are involved).

Looking in the ear one may notice a black, brown, yellow, white, or even greenish material in the ears. Sometimes, they may be relatively clean but they appear red and inflamed. Sometimes they have both a discharge and severe inflammation. In some cases, they are raw and appear extremely painful. The odor is often so strong as to make one reel backwards. **Fig. 11**

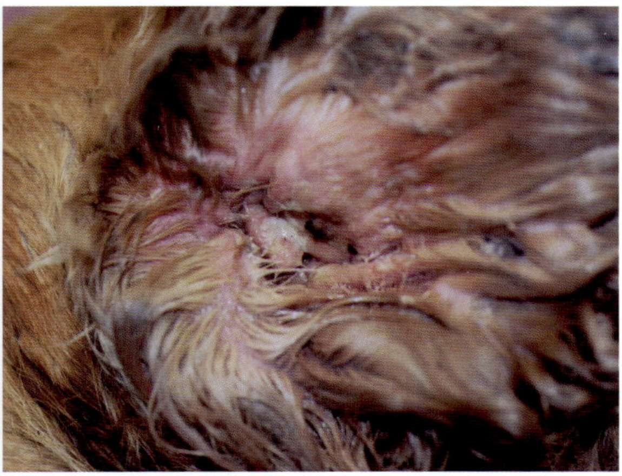

Fig. 11. A badly infected ear. Redness and odor are the two most characteristic signs.

What causes this and what can we do about it? When is it time to seek professional help? There are a variety of causes for ear infections. Allergies, water in the ears (either from a bath or a swim), ear mites or physical abnormalities in the structure of the ear (small canals, unusual flaps of cartilage which close the ear canal to air circulation, floppy ears that do the same thing) are all potential causes for ear infections.

Regardless of the cause, treatment involves cleaning and drying the ear canal. For mild cases of ear inflammation or infection, or even as a preventative, a home remedy that works is a swimmer's ear solution. This is a mixture of white vinegar and rubbing alcohol at a mixture of 50/50. The vinegar acidifies the ear while the alcohol dries out the ear canal. Obviously, this mixture can not be used in a severely inflamed or raw ear as it would sting very much. However, it is very effective the rest of the time. Simply mix the ingredients in a plastic squeeze bottle and squirt liberally into the ear canal. After the dog is through shaking his or her head, wipe out the excess with a cotton ball. Do this once a day for three or four days, then once a week for maintenance. Certainly, if the infection appears too severe and the dog will not tolerate this treatment without becoming aggressive, a more intensive medical approach (probably professional help utilizing sedation) will be required. Furthermore, if the ears are this badly inflamed, it is unlikely that the mixture above will work. **Get that suffering dog to a veterinarian right away.** They may recommend a topical antibiotic/steroid mixture as well as an oral antibiotic. Ear cleaning with or without sedation may be recommended right away or else the veterinarian may choose to allow the antibiotics to work for a week before sedation and ear flushing. Often, a maintenance solution may be recommended after this period.

One of the recent tricks that is working very well is the use of a disinfectant in the ears at a dilution that will not be toxic to the ears. Diluted chlorhexidine (diluted down to 0.25% with water) flushed into the ears daily followed by the administration of a topical antibiotic is now considered the best way to control severe ear infections. We have had success with a combination of an antibiotic known as Baytril® (enrofloxacin) small animal injectable with dexamethazone (2 mg/ml) injectable. We mix 2 ml of enrofloxacin with 3 ml of dexamethazone and 9 ml of saline solution together and apply to the ear daily for a week. The results have been very satisfactory.

Swelling of the ear is usually due to blood in the ear. Veterinarians refer to this as a hematoma. This problem is usually secondary to an infection inside of the ear and is due to a dog violently shaking their head and rupturing the blood vessels in the ear. Left untreated, the blood clot formed will contract and shrivel the ear, which may change the dog's appearance and actually worsen the air flow into the ear, increasing the risk for further infections. First aid may include bandaging the ear to the top of the head and getting that dog to a veterinarian as soon as possible. They will sedate your dog and place several holes in that ear to allow it to drain. Small hematomas may sometimes be managed by draining them with a needle and then injecting with a steroid. However, this may only work with very small hematomas or it may not work at all. The sooner this problem is treated the better. Remember that the underlying ear infection must also be treated. *This problem is also discussed in the section on lumps and bumps*. **Fig. 12**

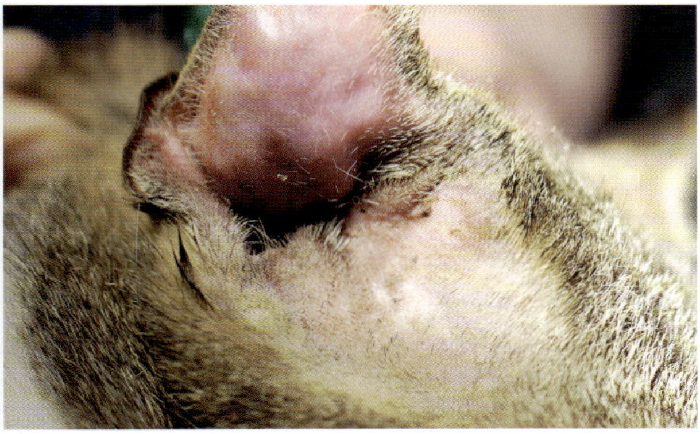

Fig. 12. Hematoma. A blood pocket forms in the ear when the head is shaken repeatedly. If not treated, it will often result in a shriveled shrunken ear that becomes chronically infected.

Lacerations in the tips of the ears may bleed profusely. First aid involves bandaging the ears to the top of the head and getting your dog to the veterinarian right away. *See the section on bleeding for a further discussion.*

Redness and rashes inside of the ear are usually due to an infection in the ear. Address the problem as discussed above.

Hair loss around the tip or margin of the ear with crusting of that area may be associated with mites (Sarcoptic mange), fly bites, or occasionally seborrhea. A number of topicals may be helpful and these may often be found over the counter in feed stores.

Keep in mind that there is often an underlying cause for chronic ear inflammation. Allergies to food or other things in the environment may be to blame. Consult your veterinarian.

Deafness is most likely due to either an acute or chronic ear infection. Sometimes wax or debris buildup may be the cause of hearing loss. As dogs age, hearing loss seems to occur just as it does in some people. Other causes may be possible but none of these may be diagnosed at home. Thus, get that dog to a veterinarian when you can. Cleaning out the ears should be the first first aid that you administer.

Eye Problems

Injuries to the eye are almost all emergencies and professional help should usually be sought immediately. First aid for a traumatized eye would include keeping the eye moist with a saline solution until it can be seen by a veterinarian. These saline eye drops can be purchased over the counter in almost any pharmacy. However, immediate professional medical treatment is often critical if an eye is to be saved.

Cloudiness on the surface of the eye or inside the eye might represent a problem as well as visible trauma to the eye. Cloudiness or a "blue" discoloration on the surface may represent corneal edema, which means that there may be an infection in front of the eye. Cloudiness inside the eye may mean that there are an increased number of cells inside of the eye. This may be either due to an infection or possibly tumor cells. If no help is available right away, a topical ophthalmic antibiotic (without any steroid) may be used three times a day until the dog can be seen by a veterinarian. Cloudiness inside of the eye may also be a cataract. These may occur from an infection or trauma, but poor diets may also contribute to them. Many are considered genetic. They tend to be progressive and generally lead to blindness. However, veterinary opthamologists may remove them surgically. Sometimes an older dog will develop a "blue haze" cloudiness of the eyes that does not seem to interfere with vision. This is called lenticular sclerosis and is an aging change that does not require treatment. However, a veterinary opthamologist may be consulted, and sometimes human eye vitamin supplements may be helpful. **Fig. 13**

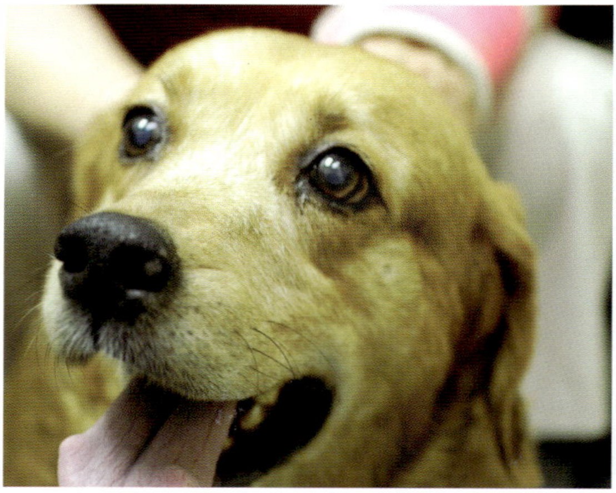

Fig. 13. Lenticular sclerosis. A clouding of the eye usually seen in older dogs.

A discharge from the eye usually suggests that an infection or an allergy is present. A general rule of thumb is that a colored discharge (green or yellow usually) is more likely to represent an infection, while a clear discharge (watery) may represent an allergy. Topical antibiotics combined with oral antibiotics will often clear an infection, while a topical containing a steroid like dexamethazone plus an oral antihistamine like Benadryl® may help solve the allergy. Of course, everything listed here except the Benadryl® is a prescription drug and they will require that a veterinarian examines the eyes and diagnoses the problem. Older dogs are more likely to develop a discharge than younger dogs, since they often lose the aqueous portion of their tears, which leaves the thicker mucous portion of the tears. This portion may contribute to a bacterial overgrowth. The treatment is to regularly apply an artificial tear solution to the eyes of an older dog, usually twice daily. Sometimes an eye discharge regularly flows onto the face and stains the area under the eyes. This is called epiphora, and it usually occurs in small breed dogs. In many cases, this is due to a blockage of the duct from the eye to the nose. A veterinarian should be consulted. **Fig. 14**

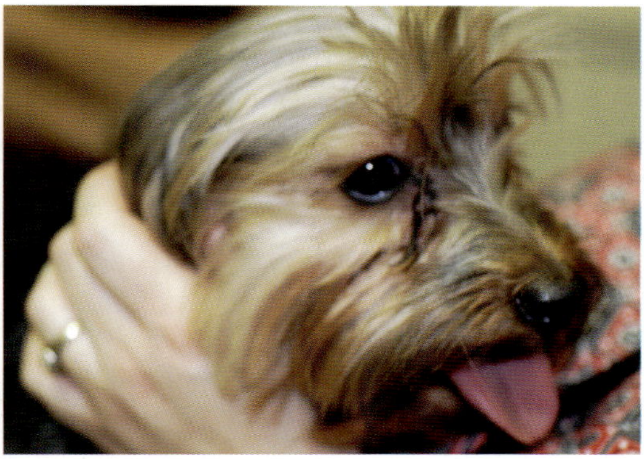

Fig. 14. Discharge from eye (epiphora). This discharge is usually created by a faulty nasolacrimal duct, which usually drains the excess tears into the nose. When the duct is either blocked by inflammation, infection or a congenital defect, it drains onto the surface of the eyelid.

A near total loss of tear production may occur in some dogs. This may result in extreme redness and inflammation as the eye becomes very dry. This is referred to as "dry eye" and it must be diagnosed by a veterinarian before you simply add artificial tears to the eye(s). However, that is exactly what you can do to provide relief until a veterinarian can be seen. The official name for this problem is keratoconjunctivitis sicca (KCS) and if you self-diagnose and treat for this without actually measuring tear production, you may actually be missing other serious problems that mimic these signs. Therefore, you must see a veterinarian.

A red discoloration in the eye may mean that there is blood in the eye. Get that dog to a veterinarian right away. Redness around the eye could suggest that there is either hemorrhage or inflammation in the tissues around the eye. This may not be as serious as blood in the eye, but it still warrants an immediate trip to the veterinarian as soon as possible. This is called conjunctivitis and it may or may not be associated with injury or infection to the eye itself. **Fig. 15**

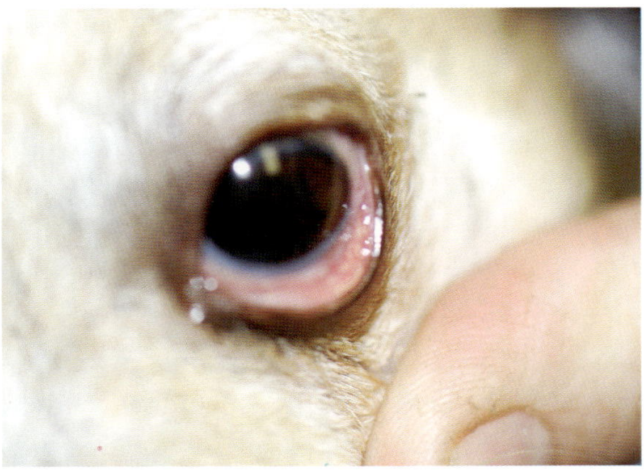

Fig. 15. Conjunctivitis/scleritis. The tissue around the eyes may become inflamed when they are exposed to either irritants or allergens.

An injury seen more commonly in short faced "brachycephalic" breeds (Pekingese, Pugs, Shih Tzus, etc... is an eye actually "popping out". This is called proptosis. If this occurs, cover the eye with a moistened paper towel and get that dog to a veterinarian right away. Time is of the essence. If the eye is still moist and viable, it may be replaced and in many cases actually retain full function! But the longer the eye is out, the greater both the drying and circulatory damage become, and the likelihood for saving the eye is minimized.

Very young puppies that have not even opened their eyes for the first time may actually develop an eye infection. This is often recognized by swelling of the eyes and a seeping of pus from a corner. The name for this is neonatal opthalmitis. If this is seen, the eyelids must be teased open and an ophthalmic antibiotic ointment must be applied or permanent damage to the eyes may occur. This procedure is often best performed by a veterinarian who may also prescribe an oral antibiotic and administer an injectable antibiotic. **Fig. 16**

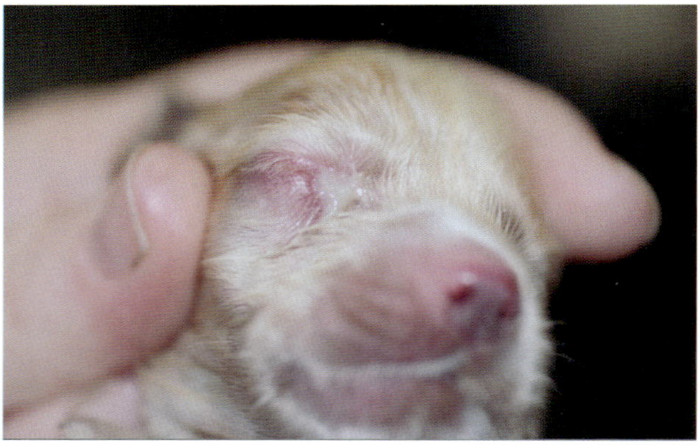

Fig. 16. Neonatal opthalmitis. An eye infection may occurs in young puppies before they even open their eyes for the first time.

Sudden blindness may occur sometimes. It may be temporary if it has occurred just following a seizure. However, a variety of other causes are possible including retinal detachment or retinal deterioration. A recently recognized syndrome known as SARDS (Sudden Acute Retinal Degeneration) has been observed in overweight dogs that may have some degree of liver disease. Inflammation of the optic nerve due to infection, trauma, or toxicity may also cause sudden blindness. You may test for blindness by moving your finger towards the eye and watching for a blink response. Some of these cases may be reversible, but none can be diagnosed or treated at home. **Get your dog to the veterinarian, or even better, a veterinary opthamologist right away.** Time is critical in cases of acute blindness.

Lumps or bumps on the eyelids could represent cysts or tumors. Have them removed fairly soon since the longer you wait, the more of the eyelid will have to be removed when surgery is finally performed. These tumors are usually glandular tumors called adenomas, and they are usually benign. **Fig. 17**

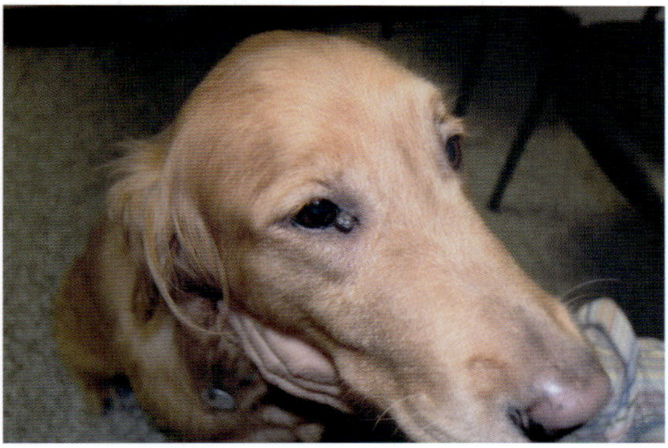

Fig. 17. Tumor on eyelid. Small tumors are common on the eyelids of older dogs. Most are benign but they should be removed regardless.

A red lump that appears inside the eye towards the side nearest to the nose is an inflammation of the gland of the third eyelid. This is called "cherry eye". It is probably an allergic reaction to something in the environment. Sometimes they can be managed medically, but most of the time they will require surgery. See your veterinarian right away since early medical intervention may help to avoid the need for surgery. The longer you wait, the more likely surgery will be necessary. **Fig. 18**

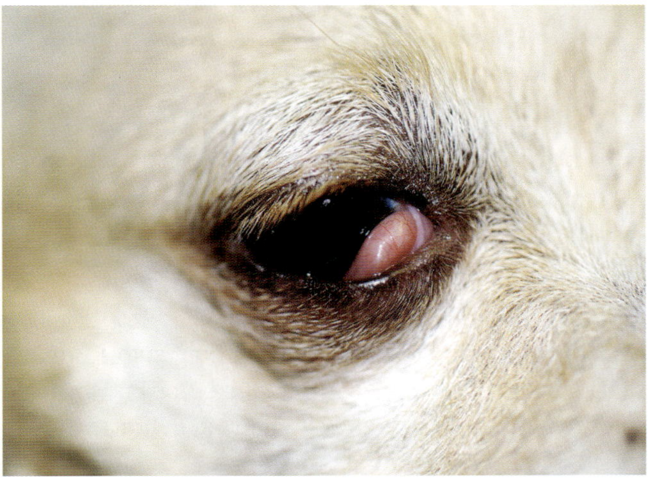

Fig. 18. Cherry eye. This is an inflammation of the gland of the third eyelid. Early treatment may clear this up but surgery is usually required.

Squinting, or eye spasms usually indicate a painful eye. In some cases, there may be a foreign object in the lid or eye itself. Often, the surface of the eye, called the cornea has been scratched. Occasionally, the surface becomes ulcerated by something irritating, including in some cases the eyelid itself. In these situations, the eyelid may be turned inward and it may be rubbing against the eye. Painful spasms of the lid may occur. First aid should include flushing the eye with a sterile eyewash or even water as soon as possible. If you can see a small object, sometimes it can be removed with a cotton tipped applicator. If there is no response, get that dog to a veterinarian right away. Objects that are imbedded probably should be removed by a veterinarian. **Fig. 19**

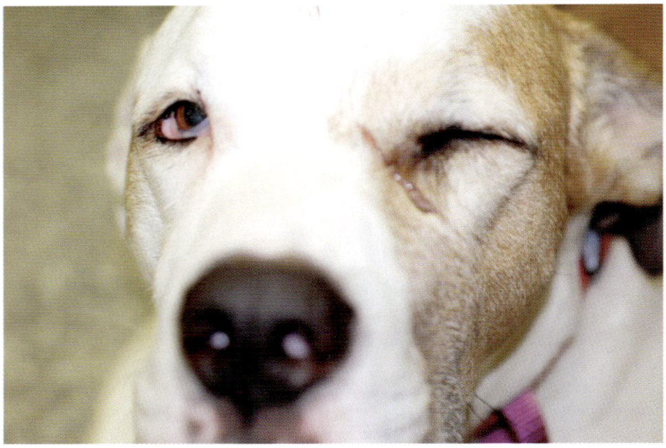

Fig. 19. Squinting/ blepharospasms. A painful eye will often result in squinting and spasming of the lid.

Bulging of the eye may suggest that there is an infection behind the eye, or rarely, the muscles around the eye. Glaucoma (increased pressure inside the eye) can also cause this. These situations must be treated by a veterinarian.

Sinking of the eye into the socket usually occurs when the fat pads behind the eyes shrink due to starvation or severe dehydration. Sometimes there is nerve or muscle damage. These situations need to be diagnosed and treated by a veterinarian.

Dilated pupils can suggest temporary or permanent damage to the brain. In acute situations, swelling of the brain is usually suspected. **Cover your pet and get it to the veterinarian right away.**

First Aid for Miscellaneous Problems

This book is organized by signs not diagnoses. However, these common problems are easily recognized (diagnosed) or known from the history of the dog. These include burns (and smoke inhalation), drowning, electric cord bite, frostbite, heat stroke, hypothermia, insect bites (with or without anaphylactic shock), and snake bites. Some of these problems have been discussed elsewhere in this book but are summarized here to improve their rapid access in an emergency situation.

Burns and Smoke Inhalation

Burns are usually easily recognized and confirmed by the known events in the area from which the dog was rescued. Ventral surfaces, particularly the feet and toes are usually affected. Redness (first degree), blisters (second degree), or charring (third degree) are all possible. Immediate first aid involves irrigating the area with room temperature clean water. One may do this for a half hour or more if the dog will tolerate it. Irrigating much longer than this may contribute to hypothermia. Irrigating the wound with dilute vinegar (1 part vinegar to 10 parts water) is an excellent alternative to water since it has excellent antibacterial activity. Then apply a topical antibiotic and consider bandaging, but keep in mind that the bandage may do more harm than good if placed too tightly. It is often better to lightly bandage and get your dog to the veterinarian. They will often sedate burned dogs to apply bandages after further irrigation of the burned areas. **Fig. 20**

Fig. 20. Burn. Redness and hair loss are the usual signs of mild burns. This was a severe burn that took three months to heal.

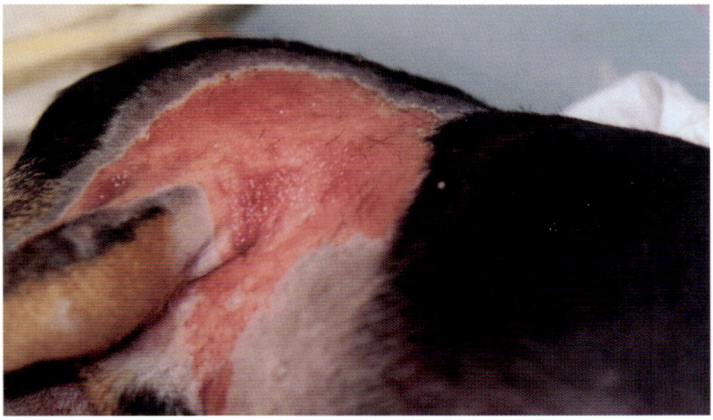

The topical of choice for burns is probably silver sulfadiazine (Silvidine®) cream. **Do not apply ice to wounds. This will worsen the injury! Make sure the body temperature is stabilized and transport to a veterinarian immediately**. If the body temperature is greater than 104°F, heat exhaustion or stroke may be present. See the heat stroke discussion below.

Smoke inhalation often accompanies a burn, and is often recognized by coughing, wheezing or rapid breathing. Sometimes the only sign will be redness around the eyes and cloudiness of the eyes. If there is a cough it is usually severe, moist and persistent. Get that dog into fresh air and to a veterinarian right away. The effects of smoke inhalation may not manifest themselves completely for hours or days after the actual inhalation, but the sooner the dog is seen and treated, the better chance it has for survival. Antibiotics, IV fluids, and bronchodilating agents may be recommended. Steroids, such as prednisilone two or three times daily are often advisable. The dose is in the drug chart.

If carbon monoxide has been involved, the gums may appear very red, even if lung damage is so severe that the gums would otherwise be blue! **These animals need to be receiving oxygen therapy right away.**

The effects of burns and smoke inhalation are far reaching and deadly. They affect nearly every system of the body, including the kidneys, intestinal tract, and immune system, not just the skin and the lungs! **Aside from rinsing off the burns, do not attempt to treat burns and smoke inhalation at home! Seek professional help! Early surgical debridement may be the best treatment and may save your dogs life. Wrap your dog up and get him to the veterinarian immediately.**

Drowning

Unable to get out of water soon enough, a dog may aspirate water into the lungs. If enough water has been aspirated to interfere with oxygen uptake, the dog will become unconscious, and then die. Prior to this point, a dog will be conscious but the fluid in the lungs will still be likely to cause significant damage to the lung tissue, and result in a severe and often fatal infection at some point in the near future.

If a dog is unconscious, remove the dog from the water, hold it upside down and allow water to drain from the lungs. One may then squeeze the abdomen in an attempt to drive more fluid from the lungs and possibly dislodge a foreign object in the trachea. Then lay the dog on its right side and massage the chest with your hands. *See the section on CPR*. For a large dog use both hands, one over the other, in short, forceful thrusts. For small dogs, you may use the thumb and forefinger on each side of the chest in the same manner. A large dog will be difficult to breathe for, however you can try to do this by forming a cone with your hand around the closed mouth and blowing into the dogs nose. For a small dog, you may place the nose and mouth in your mouth to attempt to blow air into the lungs. The head should be extended for this process (i.e. The neck must be straight) and the tongue should be pulled as far forward as you can. If breathing starts, transport the dog to a veterinarian right away. They will administer oxygen, a diuretic and antibiotics right away. Obviously, a dog that is still conscious may still need the latter treatment from a veterinarian, even if they never needed to receive CPR.

Electric Cord Bite

If a puppy suddenly develops rapid and difficult breathing, check the mouth for a blanched or scalded area across the tongue or gums. This may indicate an electric cord bite. It is possible that fluid called pulmonary edema is building up in the lungs, and this is an emergency. Get that puppy to a veterinarian immediately. They will administer a diuretic and probably oxygen. In some cases, there may be heart damage, and this will only be detectable by a veterinarian, who will detect an irregularity in the heartbeat, called a cardiac arrhythmia.

Frostbite

Frostbite is the damage caused by the freezing of tissues. In dogs, the tips of the ears and the toes are most commonly affected. It can be recognized often by white, stiff tissue. First aid includes warming the affected areas with warm water. Do not rub the area as this may tear damaged tissue. Warming these tissues may be painful, so aspirin or some other non-steroidal anti-inflammatory may be required at the dose listed in the drug chart.

Keep in mind that demarcation of the necrotic area may take days to occur. This tissue will either slough or may be removed, and the viable tissue exposed may be managed as an open wound. This means keeping the wound clean and allowing the skin to grow together over the surface. In severe cases, amputation may be required. Antibiotics should be administered to prevent infection in most cases.

Heat Stroke

While the official definition of heat stroke in people is defined as a body temperature of greater than 105° F, this is not necessarily a biologically significant temperature point for a dog. However, any temperature above 105° F accompanied by a loss of balance, disorientation and possibly rapid breathing should be considered a heat stroke type event. First aid involves immediate cooling with running cool water and possibly alcohol rub downs. Do not give water orally if these signs are present because vomiting is likely until the temperature is brought down by other means. Take the temperature regularly until it drops below 103° F and stays there. Observe for improvement in balance and mentation (alertness). If a dog can drink without vomiting, this is a sign that suggests recovery. If sterile fluids are available, they should be administered subcutaneously at the time of the initial treatment. Even if the temperature is stabilized, the dog should be taken to a veterinarian as soon as possible. Steroids like dexamethazone and antibiotics may be helpful in cases of heat stroke and its sequelae.

Hypothermia

The opposite of heat stroke is hypothermia. A low body temperature of less than 98° F is suggestive of hypothermia in a dog. This occurs when a dog is unable to generate enough heat to maintain its body temperature. The dog may be shivering and stumbling. In severe cases, they may actually appear dead, with very slow breathing and little or no movement. First aid involves rapid warming in any way possible. A dog that appears frozen without a heartbeat should only receive the breathing part of CPR as described above. Cardiac massage may trigger a fatal cardiac rhythm. Warmed sterile fluids may be administered subcutaneously if they are available. Take the temperature regularly until it returns to normal (approximately 100-102° F). **Get that dog to a veterinarian immediately.** They will treat for shock and the likely sequelae to hypothermia. If there are any signs of frostbite, treat as discussed above.

Insect bites (or stings) with or without anaphylactic shock

Insect bites or stings may be associated with a severe local or systemic reaction. Admittedly, a systemic reaction does not occur with every bite or sting, but if it occurs, it is very serious. This systemic reaction is referred to as anaphylactic shock, and if left untreated, it may be fatal. First aid for a bite or sting involves washing the area of the bite or sting with soap and water or surgical scrub. Use needle nose pliers or forceps to remove the stinger if it can be seen. Apply hydrocortisone cream topically to the site. Give diphenhydramine capsules or liquid (Benadryl®) orally at the dose listed in the drug chart (2 mg/kg or 1 mg/lb). If anaphylactic shock is occurring, it will be manifested by swelling around the mouth and throat, rapid breathing, wheezing, vomiting, and sometimes diarrhea (and it may be bloody).

Treatment of anaphylactic shock would include the treatment listed above for the bite, plus the use of epinephrine injectable at the dose listed in the drug chart (approximately .02 cc/kg or .01 cc per pound of body weight) given subcutaneously. If successful, the swelling and difficult breathing will often improve within 15 minutes. If not, be prepared to administer more diphenhydramine and epinephrine within 30 minutes. A veterinarian may also administer a steroid such as dexamethazone IV or IM at a dose of 2 mg/kg (1 mg/lb). **Get that dog to a veterinarian right away if possible.**

Make sure that you keep diphenhydramine on hand for possible future anaphylactic events. Even if your dog has never had such an event occur, this drug is a life saver! Keep some on hand at all times. This agent and epinephrine containing syringes are present in anaphylactic shock kits, which are available over the counter.

Snake Bite

A venomous snake bite by a viper (Rattlesnakes, Copperheads, Cottonmouths in North America, or Adders in Europe) is usually manifested by the presence of a draining puncture wound. One or two punctures may be present, and the drainage is usually bloody. The tissue around the puncture may be swollen, and the tissue right at the puncture site may be turning black. The vast majority of snake bites in dogs are on the snout or side of the face. Left untreated, severe swelling around the head and neck may impede breathing, or circulatory compromise may occur. Either or both of these events may result in death. Bitten dogs are usually restless at first, but then become lethargic. **See Vet ASAP!**

First aid includes keeping your dog calm and confining it until it can be transported to the veterinarian. Antihistamines such as diphenhydramine (Benadryl®) may be given orally at a dose of 2 mg/kg (1 mg/lb). Most other measures, including incision and sucking out venom are ineffective. Applying ice is not considered very helpful either. One may wash the wound with cool water, but do not use soap as this may increase the venom absorption. Antibiotics, fluids and anti-inflammatory pain medications are usually indicated. Antivenin may be recommended by a veterinarian.

The bite from an elapid snake (coral snakes, cobras, mambas) tends not to swell much but the venom of such snakes acts upon the nervous system and usually causes death by paralysis of the diaphragm (the large muscle that controls breathing). Dogs bitten by coral snakes will become progressively weaker and have difficulty swallowing. Antivenin and assisted respiration may be required in order to save animals bitten by these snakes. The major effects of such a venom usually start within an hour and last for 3 to 5 days, while those of a viper bite (tissue damage) begin immediately and may last for months or longer. Sometimes muscle or nerve damage is permanent.

Flaking Skin

Flaky skin is a common problem in dogs. It usually seems to occur in dogs that have other underlying problems, such as parasites, allergies, or infections. Eliminate the external parasites by utilizing one of the modern flea control agents. Consider a food trial for several weeks with a hypoallergenic diet. Consult with your veterinarian about the possibility of an infection with bacteria or yeast. You may try an antibacterial shampoo initially but often oral antibiotics are necessary.

A number of over the counter products have been helpful in reducing flaky skin. These include fish oil capsules and the other omega fatty acid supplements. Follow the label directions.

Sometimes flaking is associated with a disease process known as primary seborrhea. This is a condition which is not entirely understood, but it involves the abnormal production of oils in the skin. Sometimes there is not enough. Sometimes, there is too much. This problem may be heritable and can be very difficult to control. Seek professional help if the problem is persistent.

Internal parasites often rob nutrients from dogs, and one of these manifestations may be flaky skin. Have your dog checked for worms or perform a routine deworming if you can't see the veterinarian right away.

Fleas, Ticks and other Creepy Crawlers

Fleas are the most common parasite of dogs. They cause irritation, itching (pruritis), hair loss, and anemia. Furthermore, they are the major vector for tapeworms in dogs. They are a major cause of allergic reactions in dogs and their bites may lead to infections of the skin as well. At the very least, they make dogs miserable. **Left untreated, they can kill a dog!**

Perhaps the most common sign observed with fleas is scratching and chewing. Often this results in hair loss, and the most common pattern is a loss on the rump and down the back of the rear legs. If this pattern is observed, fleas must be suspected! Strangely, many owners have no idea their dog has fleas, and when advised that they do, they don't believe it. I have referred to this as FDS (Flea Denial Syndrome). While this is meant to be somewhat humorous, the results are not. Dogs whose owners don't treat their fleas will suffer needlessly.

Flea control products have become very effective in recent years. Interestingly, while they have become more effective, they have also become safer. These products include Advantage®, Comfortis®, Frontline®, Revolution® and others. However, I would like to add a word of warning. There are some products out there that are not particularly effective or especially safe. Use one of those listed above and you will generally be satisfied with the results. Keep in mind that although these products are generally marketed to apply once monthly, it may be better to apply them every three weeks if you are experiencing difficulties. The flea life cycle is three weeks. Thus using these products every three weeks may help to increase their effectiveness. **Fig. 21**

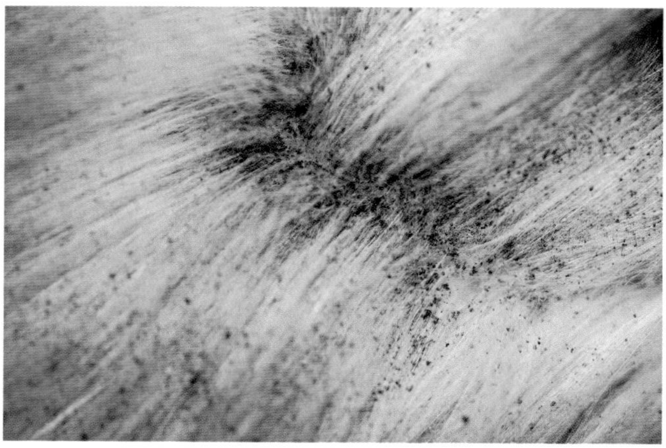

Fig. 21. Fleas and flea dirt (flea feces). Most of the newer products to control fleas are safe, but must be applied regularly in order to be effective.

Ticks are not fleas! While this may seem like a ridiculous statement, the truth is evident if you have ever had to deal with a tick infestation. Keep in mind that 99% of the tick population lives off of the dog and that they can live for two years without a meal. Add to this that ticks can hibernate through very cold winters and that they are active most of the year, and you have a real parasitic nightmare. Furthermore, some species can survive and reproduce inside of a house! **Fig. 22**

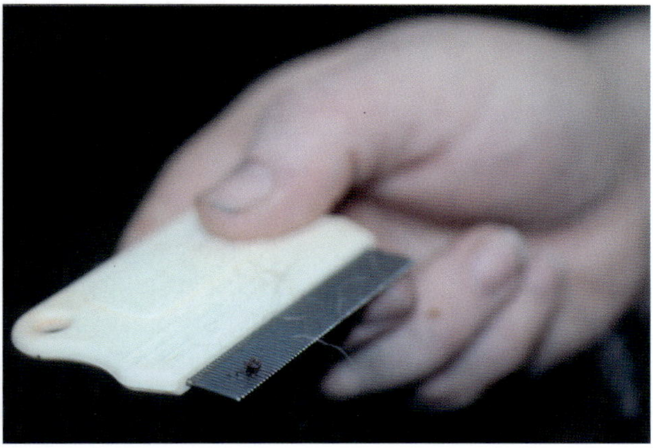

Fig. 22. Ticks. Ticks are very difficult to eliminate because they spend 95% of their life off of the dog. Thus the environment needs to be treated as well.

Several topicals exist that kill ticks. These include Advantix®, Frontline®, Promeris®, and Vectra®. Most are over 95% effective at killing ticks on the dog. However, even a small number of live ticks on your dog are obvious. Therefore, you don't believe that the products work. They are working, but you may need professional help to control the tick population in your yard and home, since as mentioned above, most of them are not on your dog and they do not reproduce on your dog!

Fractures

First aid for fractures often involves immobilizing a bone with an obvious angular displacement or a lack of support (a dangling limb). Since many dogs are resistant to manipulating their injured limbs, it often makes more sense to keep them confined and get them to professional help as soon as possible. One may administer pain medication such as aspirin, Rimadyl® or Metacam® at the dose listed in the drug chart. Thus, confinement and pain relief are the best options prior to seeing a veterinarian. With a compound fracture (if the bone is sticking out or there is a major tear in the skin at the site of the fracture suggesting that a bone has been exposed temporarily), irrigate the wound with saline solution and apply a topical and oral antibiotic if they are available, and immediate veterinary care is not available. **Fig. 23**

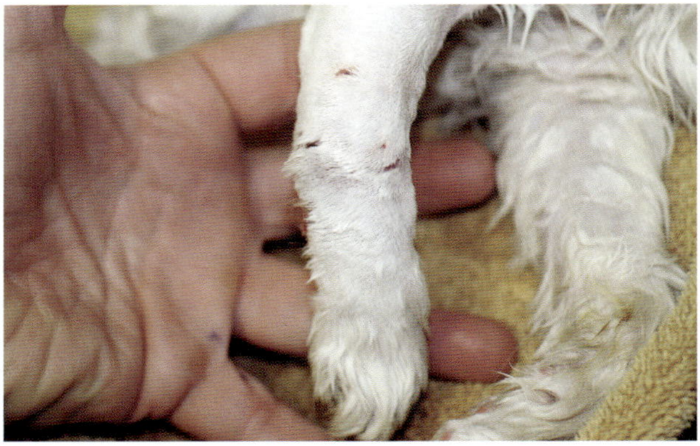

Fig. 23. Fracture/angular displacement. The abnormal angle of this foot indicates a fracture.

Only attempt splinting if help is not immediately available and check the area carefully to look for signs of poor circulation (blueness, coolness, or swelling) once a splint has been applied. If these signs are seen, the splint may have to be removed or loosened. Seeing these signs in an unbandaged, unsplinted limb could suggest that the circulation has been compromised by the break and the limb may have to be straightened out immediately. It could then be splinted. Obviously, this is best performed by a veterinarian who will administer anesthesia and analgesia during this process.

Frothing at the Mouth

The most common reason for frothing at the mouth in dogs is the recent ingestion of something noxious or irritating. This may include poisonous plants, toads, or chemicals. First aid usually involves rinsing the mouth out with copious quantities of water from the garden hose. One may then wish to transport the pet to a veterinarian for further care and possible administration of an antidote.

Other things that may cause frothing would be nausea, a dental infection, a tongue or mouth injury, difficulty swallowing, or electrical burns in the mouth from chewing on an electrical cord.

While this description often engenders visions of a rabid raccoon or fox, this is very rare. It is much less common than the ingestion of a substance as described above. If a medicine has just been administered and frothing is observed, one may wish to rinse the mouth out with some water.

If frothing at the mouth is associated with any neurological signs however, such as muscle tremors or weakness in the rear legs, or a change in behavior, then there is a greater likelihood for rabies. Only about one third of dogs affected by rabies become aggressive. Keep in mind that an animal can only catch rabies from exposure to a wild carnivore or a bat that has the disease. Furthermore, infection with the rabies virus requires a bite from one of those animals.

If rabies is suspected, a veterinarian may recommend hospitalization and observation if the signs are mild, or euthanasia if the signs are advanced. A definitive diagnosis cannot be determined in a live animal.

Hair Loss (Circles, Patches and Patterns)

One of the most obvious signs of a dermatological problem in the dog is hair loss. Veterinarians recognize several patterns of hair loss and can usually determine the cause. These causes include food allergies, flea allergies, contact allergies, and inhalant allergies (atopy). Several types of mange and fungus may cause hair loss as well. Other signs are often associated with hair loss. These include redness (erythema), itching (pruritis), flaking, and various signs of infection. Long term hair loss may be associated with graying of the skin (hyperpigmentation) and thickening of the skin (hyperkeratosis). One of the common names for this combination is "elephant skin". **Fig. 24**

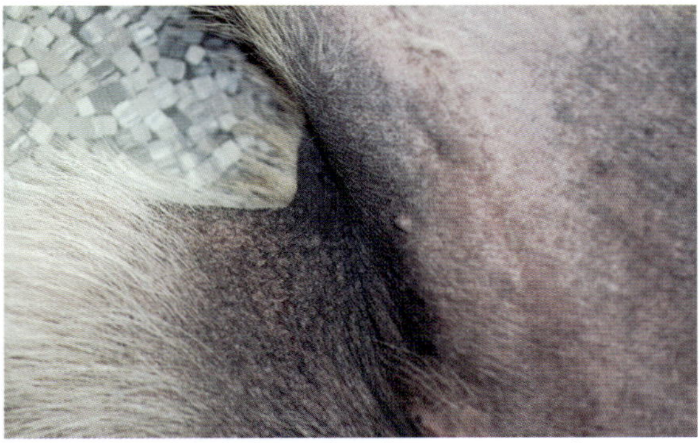

Fig. 24. Hair loss/redness/hyperpigmentation/hyperkeratosis (elephant skin). Any chronic irritation will result in redness first, followed by hyperpigmentation and then thickening.

A pattern of hair loss that is most prominent on the rump and back of the legs is a flea allergy pattern. Administer flea control as recommended in the section on fleas. **Fig. 25**

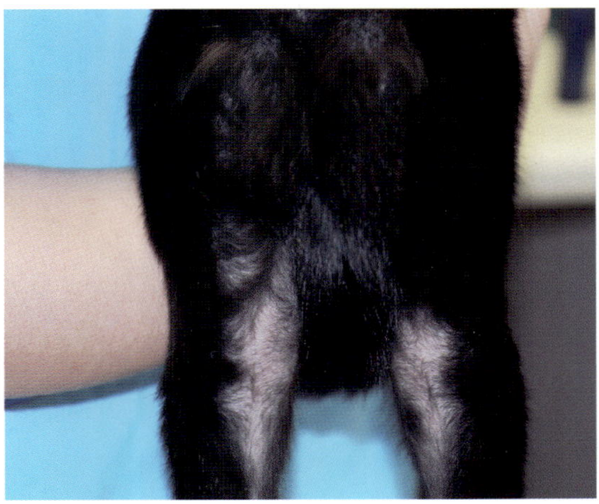

Fig. 25. FAD (Flea Allergy Dermatitis). Hair loss on the rump and down the back of the rear legs is often suggestive of a flea allergy dermatitis.

A pattern of hair loss that is between the toes and on the chest and belly (abdomen) is usually a contact allergy, or possibly just exposure to an irritant in the environment over a prolonged period of time. Examine the environment and the dog's behavior patterns. If your pet is spending a lot of time on the grass, one might suspect an allergy to the grass or some chemical on the grass. If spending a lot of time on a carpet, suspect the carpet itself or a cleaner used on the carpet. Generally speaking, cleansers or detergents that are scented are more likely to cause allergic reactions. For this problem, one may change carpets or cleansers and see if there is a response. If not, see a veterinarian. You can not totally rule out a food allergy however. **Fig. 26**

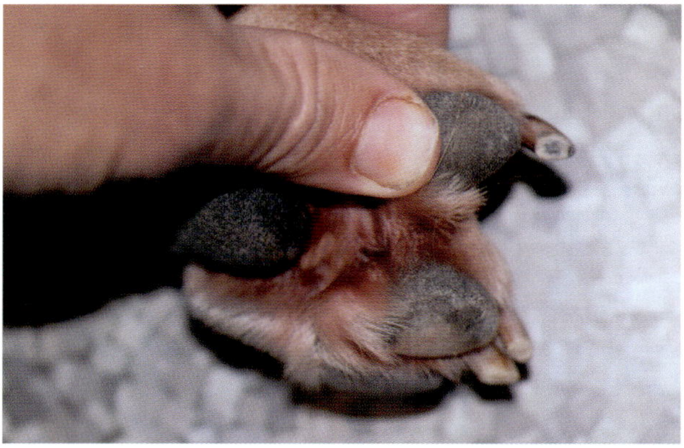

Fig. 26. Redness between toes can occur because of a contact allergy or a food allergy. It may also be due to a burn or exposure to some irritant.

A pattern of hair loss that is everywhere (generalized) and usually associated with redness, even in the ears, is probably an inhalant allergy (atopy). The eyes may also be red (conjunctivitis). There are only two options here since gas masks are not practical for dogs. These include moving out of your house (or state) or more practically have your dog tested for allergens by your veterinarian. Once the allergens are known, a dog can be hyposensitized by a series of specially prepared vaccines. Short term relief may involve the use of antihistamines or steroids or cyclosporine (Atopica®). **Fig. 27**

Fig. 27. Atopy is the name that dermatologists use for an allergy to something "in the air". It has been referred to as "inhalant dermatitis" but this term has fallen into disfavor since the allergen does not have to be inhaled. Lesions are usually widely distributed. Ears are often red to the tips, and both the skin and eyes also appear red and inflamed.

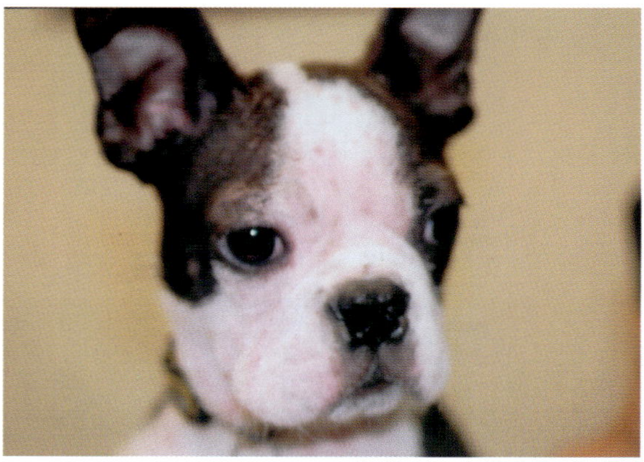

A pattern of hair loss around the eyes in a young dog (often a purebred), is usually suggestive of demodectic mange. This is a species of mite that is present in most dogs but seems to cause problems primarily in young dogs that are immunosuppressed by internal parasites, malnutrition or stress. The predisposition to show the disease is heritable, so these dogs should not be bred. Treatment for this problem can include vitamin supplements and deworming, but professional help may be required to eliminate this mite. Ivermectin may be given orally every day for one to two months or you may use a product called Mitaban® Dip once per week.

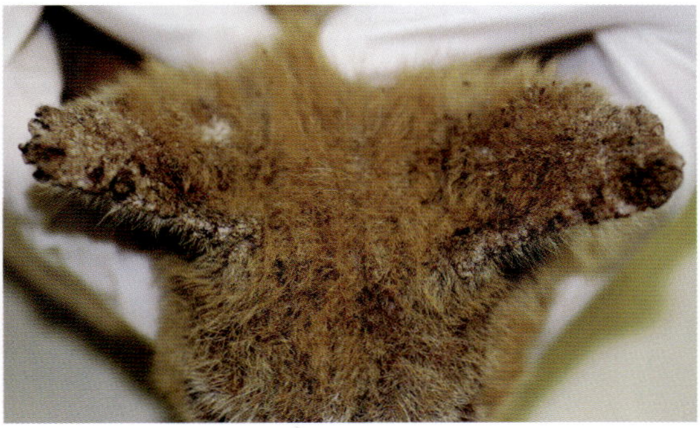

Fig. 28. Sarcoptic mange is caused by the *Sarcoptes* sp. mange mites. Note the crusty appearance. These mites are highly contagious to other animals including cats, and people. Fortunately, they are relatively easy to eliminate.

A pattern of hair loss along the edges of the ears, around the eyes and elsewhere is suggestive of sarcoptic mange. This type of mange is easier to eliminate, often requiring only two injections of ivermectin at the dose listed in the drug chart. However, it is contagious to humans and other pets. Therefore, if you see an intensely itchy dog with hair loss on the face and ears, **get that dog to a veterinarian right away. Fig. 28**

A pattern of hair loss that is circular in nature may be indicative of a fungal infection. The common name for this problem is ringworm, but this is not a worm at all, but rather a group of fungi that grow on the skin of many animals and people. They are called dermatophytes, which means "skin eaters". If there are just one or two circles present, they may be managed by applying topical miconazole once daily for about a month. Miconazole is available over the counter. Wash your hands off after touching these areas since you are susceptible to this infection as well. I also recommend shampooing the entire dog with an antifungal shampoo such as Chlorhexiderm® once per week during that month.

A single patch of missing hair that occurs suddenly that is red, moist and sometimes has a little pus on the surface is a "hot spot". The official name for this is acute moist pyotraumatic dermatitis (AMPD), and that means that it is a rapidly appearing spot associated with self trauma (chewing) that is moist and infected. The cause is often unknown, but an allergy to something is the most likely initiating factor. Cleaning the spot and applying a topical liquid hydrocortisone every few hours for 12 hours may arrest the itching and allow the spot to begin to heal. You may also give diphenhydramine HCL (Benadryl®) at a dose of 1 mg/pound (2 mg/kg) every four hours during that first 12 hours and twice per day afterwards to help control the itch. However, sometimes the itching is so intense that a veterinarian may have to administer a steroid shot to break the itch cycle and antibiotics may be required as well.

A pattern of hair loss that includes a combination of all of the above (with the exception of the two kinds of mange and ringworm) may suggest a food allergy. Review the dietary habits and consider trying a hypoallergenic diet for at least 3 weeks. Keep treats to a minimum. Seek professional advice in order to confirm this and provide the correct diet. My recommended diet of choice is Hill's Z/D®.

Interestingly, there is an old treatment that is potentially curative of both major kinds of mange, as well as lice, fleas, fungal infections, and many bacterial infections! It stinks of rotten eggs, but if you are willing to deal with the smell and use it every five days, here is the treatment...Lime Sulfur Dip! Simply mix as directed on the label and apply.

Head Tilt

A head tilt is a serious sign. It usually represents a middle ear infection on the side to which the head is tilted. Check the ears to determine if there is any inflammation visible in the external ear canal but keep in mind that there may not be any observable change in the external ear. Seek professional help right away. If professional help is not immediately available, one may administer aspirin at the dose recommended in the drug chart in order to relieve pain and discomfort. This is only to provide temporary relief until a veterinarian can be seen. Do not administer immediately prior to going to the vet, however, since this may limit the veterinarians choice of drugs at the time of treatment.

Another reason for a head tilt is a lesion in the vestibular region of the brain. This may either be infectious, traumatic or neoplastic (a tumor). These kinds of lesions are often associated with a windshield wiper-like motion in the eyes called nystagmus. The eyes rapidly move toward the side of the lesion and the head tilt. This requires immediate professional help.

Itching (Pruritis)

The causes for itching (scratching) are generally the same as they are for hair loss. These include a variety of allergies and parasites such as mites, fleas, or ticks. Dermatophytes, or skin attacking fungi may also cause itching. The allergies include food allergies, contact allergies, and atopy (inhalant or exposure allergies). See that section for a discussion of allergy treatment and parasite control. The first line of defense is removal of the offending agent. Move the dog to another area, and consider washing it off. **Adminster Benadryl® (diphenhydramine) at a dose of 2 mg/kg (1 mg/lb) twice daily or more frequently if the itching is severe. Consider using topical hydrocortisone on lesions as well.** Sometimes, severe itching will lead to more serious dermatological problems, such as acral lick granulomas, hot spots or a staph infection (pyoderma). Thus, chronic itchiness with self trauma must be treated by a veterinarian, who will often administer powerful anti-inflammatory agents called steroids as well as antibiotics, after they diagnose and eliminate the primary cause. Keep in mind that allergy testing may be recommended. Sometimes a hypoallergenic food trial may be utilized. Skin scrapings, fungal or bacterial cultures may be recommended. Be patient. Itching is not a specific sign, and diagnosis of the cause is often a process of elimination.

Home treatment of itchy skin may include twice weekly bathings with a chlorhexidine shampoo. Let it stay on for 10 minutes before rinsing. Oral supplementation with omega 3 fish oils at a dose of 800 mg per 20 kg of body weight is also likely to reduce itchiness.

One of the newer non-steroidal treatments for atopy (an absorbed/inhaled allergy) is a product called Atopica®. This effective product contains microencapsulated cyclosporine, which is an immune system suppressant. The dose is listed in the drug chart.

Lethargy

The causes for lethargy are numerous. The most common causes of lethargy include anemia, and fever, but gastrointestinal distress, toxicity and many other things are possible. This is not something that can be diagnosed at home, so **get your dog to the veterinarian right away.** First aid for lethargy involves symptomatic treatment. Oral fluids are always a good move, and sometimes a non-steroidal anti-inflammatory agent will help, such as aspirin or Rimadyl®. A veterinarian may want to perform bloodwork and even take a radiograph (X-ray) in order to determine the cause of the lethargy. Many times they will discover things that were not suspected. Thus, in cases of lethargy, you are strongly advised to get your family pet to the veterinarian right away. **Fig. 29**

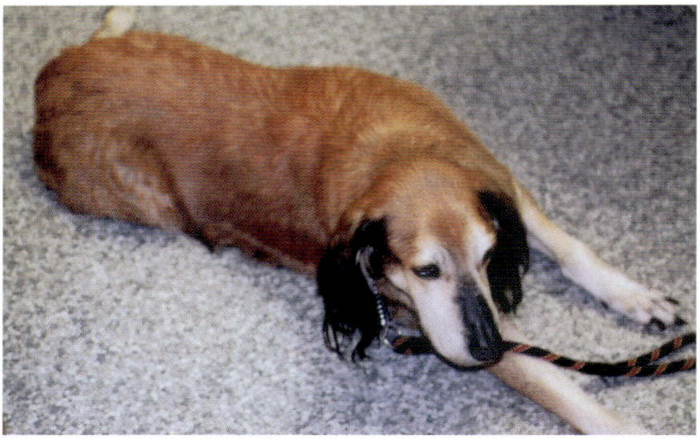

Fig. 29. Lethargic dog. Lethargy is a non-specific but very serious sign.

Licking

Licking or chewing at any area suggests pain or discomfort at that spot. Check the area carefully for insect bites or stingers. Remove these objects if visible.

Lumps and Bumps

There are many causes for lumps and bumps in a dog. Small lumps and bumps that are found widely distributed in the skin are likely to be evidence of a skin infection called pyoderma. Soft lumps seen on older dogs, particularly females, are very likely to be lipomas, or fatty tumors. Wart like structures seen in older dogs are likely to be papillomas, which are common benign tumors of older dogs. Lipomas and papillomas may be removed for cosmetic reasons, but they are not generally considered a serious threat since they are benign. The only time these tumors need to be removed immediately is if they are interfering with locomotion (as in the case of a large lipoma) or if they are bleeding (as in the case of a papilloma that has been scratched open). **Fig. 30, Fig. 31**

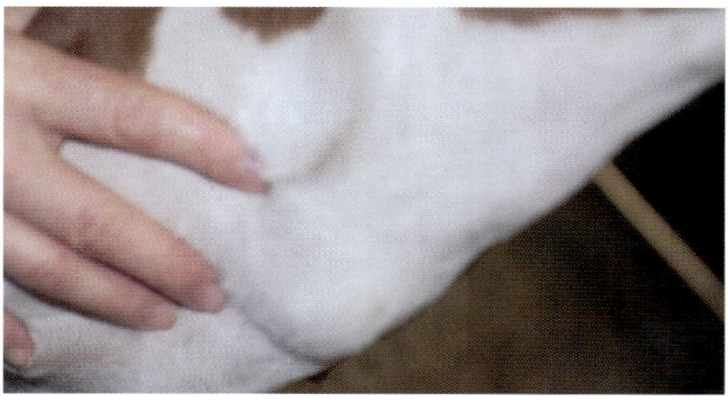

Fig. 30. Lipoma. Lipomas are fatty tumors. They are usually soft and easily moveable masses. They are benign and usually do not need to be removed unless they interfere with locomotion.

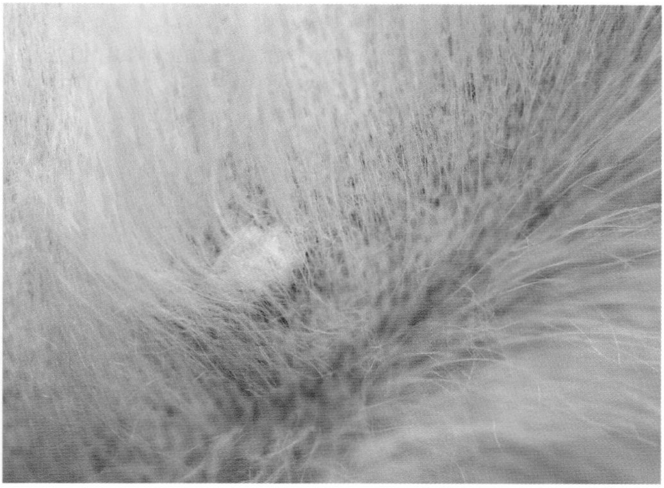

Fig. 31. Papilloma. Papilloma are virally induced tumors that are common in older dogs. They are usually removed for cosmetic reasons unless they are bleeding, in which case they should be removed immediately.

Sometimes soft lumps are not tumors at all, but sebaceous cysts, which are hollow fluid filled pockets. These cysts may eventually rupture spontaneously or they may be surgically removed. Suddenly appearing soft lumps in the abdomine are usually hernias and should be looked at by a vet as soon as possible.

Firm lumps anywhere are more serious than soft lumps and these should be removed as soon as possible and sent in for histopathology. A firm swelling that appears to involve a bone or otherwise be very firmly attached is very ominous and should be immediately examined by a veterinarian, who may choose to remove it or biopsy it. These firmly attached lumps are more likely to be aggressive tumors than those that are not well attached.

Firm lumps are not always aggressive tumors however. Sometimes they are nothing more than bruises on the surface of a bone. Keep in mind that a solid blow to the surface of a bone may initiate the same kind of bone reaction as a break, and a firm callus may occur where the trauma occurred.

One unusual manifestation of this is the lump that occurs on top of the head of a young hyperactive dog when it comes up too fast underneath a coffee table. This may fracture the ridge on top of the head known as the occipital crest. The resulting swelling is usually cone shaped, and thus I have referred to this as "conehead syndrome." Young Irish Setters and Labs appear particularly prone to this.

Sometimes, bumps may appear suddenly all over a dog. These are likely to be hives. Hives suggest that there has been a sudden allergic reaction to something in the environment. They can also occur with the consumption of a food, the administration of a medicine or the use of a topical shampoo or flea control product. Immediate first aid involves the administration of diphenhydramine

HCL (Benadryl®) at a dose of 1 mg/pound of body weight (2 mg/Kg). See the drug chart. If the hives occur after exposure to a topical product, you may also wish to wash the dog off with soap and water as well.

As mentioned above, small bumps everywhere may suggest the presence of a skin infection called pyoderma. Literally translated this means pus in the skin. Indeed, this is likely to be a bacterial infection, and in most cases it is a Staph infection. That is, it is an infection caused by a bacteria known as *Staphylococcus*. Antibiotics will be required. **Fig. 32**

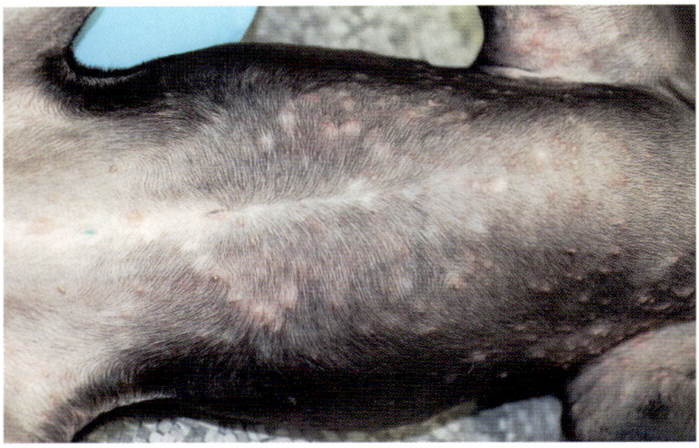

Fig. 32. Pyoderma. Literally translated, this term means "pus in the skin", and it can be recognized by pustules and papules on the skin. The bacterial infection is usually secondary to some other factor however, such as an allergy.

Bumps in or near the mammary glands may be either an infection of the mammary glands or possibly a tumor. If a young dog has recently been in heat or recently weaned puppies, there is a possibility that she has an infection called mastitis. If an older dog has firm lumps there, it is much more likely to be a mammary tumor. Sometimes a female dog may have what is called a false pregnancy. During this time a female dog may look pregnant, act pregnant, and even develop large, milk filled mammary glands, even though she is not pregnant. Antibiotics will be required to treat mastitis and an ovariohysterectomy (spaying) will probably be curative.

A firm elevated bump on the front leg that has a raw appearing top and is the target of the dog's frequent licking and chewing, is likely to be an acral lick granuloma. These are believed to be inflamed tissues secondary to an infection. They may start as an itch, but as a dog continues to chew on that spot, they become inflamed and infected. They are very difficult to eliminate, even for a veterinarian, and because some dogs become obsessive about chewing on them. Some dermatologists now believe that they are due to a food allergy. Others think that they may be due to a contact allergy. It is possible that both kinds of allergies may contribute to the problem in some cases. In any case, this is not an emergency, but get your dog to the veterinarian as soon as possible. The sooner they begin treating this, the better chance they will have to eliminate it. They may prescribe antibiotics, steroids and a dietary change. Even if the treatment is correct, it may take months to eliminate these unusual "lumps." **Fig. 33**

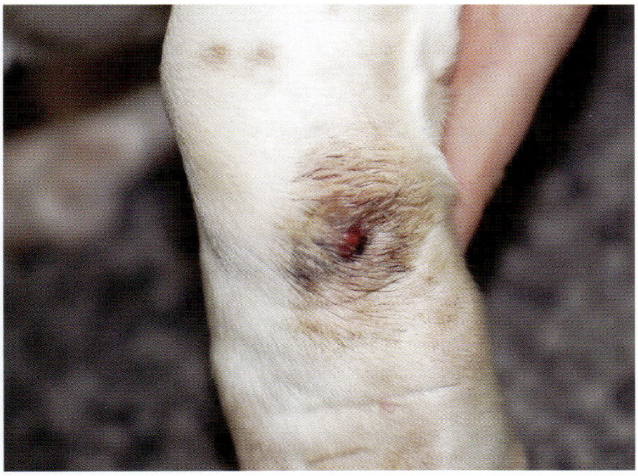

Fig. 33. Acral lick granuloma. These are one of the most difficult and frustrating dermatological problems that we see in dogs. It is believed that the underlying cause may be an allergy....probably a food allergy.

Dogs have four sets of palpable (feelable) lymph nodes. These are the submandibulars (located at the angle of the jaw and neck), the prescapulars (in front of the shoulder blades), inguinals (in the groin area), and popliteals (behind the knees). If there is an infection near one of these paired lymph nodes, they may become larger or reactive. Usually a single enlarged lymph node indicates a local infection, while multiple lymph node enlargement may represent a more ominous disease, possibly lymphoma (a cancer of the lymph system). This can not be diagnosed at home. Get your dog to the veterinarian as soon as possible. They will perform a needle aspirate or a biopsy in order to determine what is happening. Don't despair. There are protocols for chemotherapy of lymphoma that are often very effective. **Fig. 34**

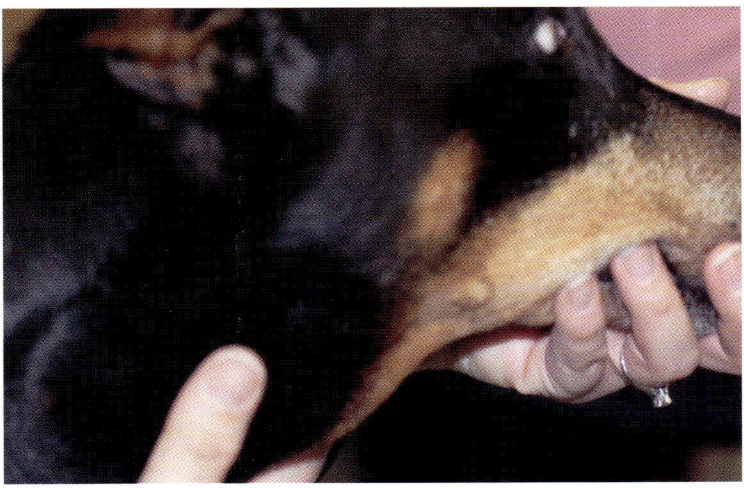

Fig. 34. Enlarged lymph node. Enlarged lymph nodes are a serious sign. They may be reactive due to a local infection or they may be harboring abnormal (cancer) cells.

Muscle Wasting

The loss of muscle mass is a frightening sign. The causes are numerous but since none may be diagnosed at home, one must consult a veterinarian. Generalized muscle wasting may be associated with kidney disease, pancreatic disease or an intestinal disorder. An autoimmune disease may also be involved. Deterioration of a single muscle may be due to nerve damage or severe joint damage. In any case, rapid diagnosis and treatment may save the muscle, or muscles involved. Seek veterinary help immediately at the earliest sign of muscle wasting.

Obesity

Some veterinarians believe that 30 – 40 % of dogs are obese, or that they weigh more than they should for their body type. Obesity in dogs has the same serious implications for the health of a dog as it does for people. Obese dogs are more prone to heart disease, diabetes, arthritis, ligament damage, tumors, slow healing, and heat intolerance. They also find it more difficult to exercise which makes the problem worse.

The first step in solving the problem is to recognize it. The easiest way to do this is look at the dog's waist. Does it have one? If the waist is larger that the chest, it is generally a sign that a dog is overweight. If you can not feel the ribs easily, your dog is probably overweight. Consult with your veterinarian if you are not sure. **Fig. 35**

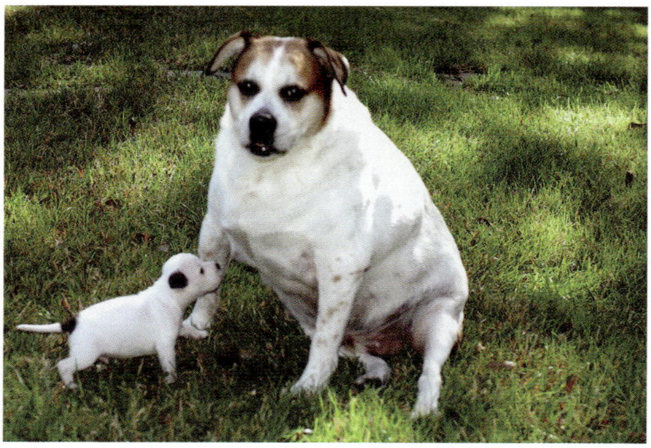

Fig. 35. Obese dog. Obesity is a very common and serious problem in pet dogs. It may predispose to joint problems, heart disease, and diabetes among other problems.

Once it has been determined that a dog is overweight, dietary changes can be implemented. There are a number of both prescription and over the counter diets that will help. In addition, an owner serious about helping his or her dog lose weight must reevaluate the kind of snacks they are giving and how many. Since snacks are just that, there is no need for their manufacturers to balance their nutritional value. To make them tasty, they are often high in fat and salt content, which is exactly what you don't want to be feeding an obese dog. One can easily compare the fat content of the snack with a dog's food in order to determine just how fattening the snack will be. Alternatives include carrots and other vegetables (but not onions), and fruits, as well as those snacks marked as "light" or lower calorie treats.

Obesity is not always due to overeating. Sometimes a slow metabolism is to blame. Hypothyroidism is an underactive thyroid gland and is the most common metabolic cause for obesity. It is often associated with other signs such as constipation, low activity, low body temperature, and dry, flaky skin. Hypothyroidism must be diagnosed by a veterinarian, who will run bloodwork in order to determine the level of thyroid hormones. Supplementation of these hormones may result in a rapid weight loss and improvement of other signs as well.

Old Dog Problems (Geriatrics)

Older dogs are prone to many of the problems that other older animals and people are prone to. These problems include muscle loss, heart disease, kidney disease, liver disease, pancreatic disease, gastroenteritis, and arthritis. In many cases, more than one system will be failing. *See the section on Behavioral Changes*. In addition, vision loss and hearing loss may occur. Bone density loss and degenerative bone disease are likely. Furthermore, older dogs are more prone to a variety of tumors. Metabolic problems such as diabetes, hypothyroidism, Addison's disease and others are also more likely. In general, older dogs are often in a state of catabolism (breakdown) instead of anabolism (build up) of muscle mass. **Fig. 36**

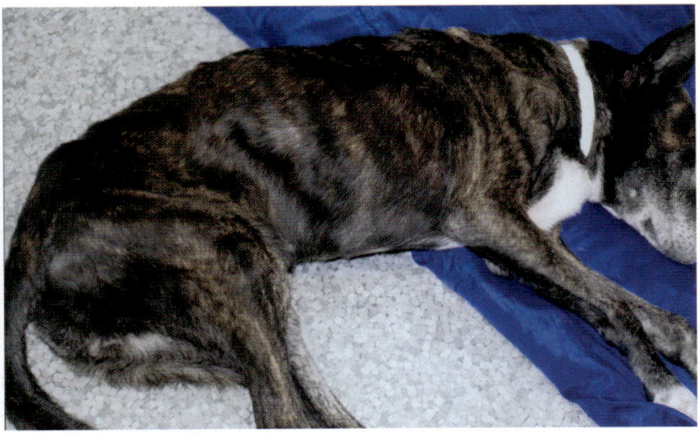

Fig. 36. Old dog (catabolic). Older dogs are often in a catabolic state. This means that they are breaking down muscle. Various foods and supplements may be helpful in reversing this.

So what does the concerned geriatric dog owner do? Firstly, have your senior dog examined every six months to a year and consider having a geriatric blood screen done at least once yearly. By the way, a dog should be considered a senior dog if it is over 8 years old, especially if it is a large breed dog.

Secondly, make sure to be feeding a good quality dog food formulated for a senior dog. There are many brands that produce such foods and label them clearly for use in older dogs.

Thirdly, consider vitamin and mineral supplements, especially if your dog is on a diuretic like furosemide (Lasix®) for heart disease. In addition, natural supplements, such as glucosamine and chondroitin are known to help maintain joint health. I often recommend creatine as well for some of my geriatric patients, in order to help them maintain or increase muscle mass. Hill's Corporation, the manufacturer of Science Diets® and Prescription Diets® actually incorporates this ingredient in some of their foods for older dogs, such as G/D® food.

Fourthly, remember the value of exercise. Regular exercise benefits all systems, including the circulatory and respiratory system as well as the joints, muscles and bones. Furthermore, its great for their attitude. Take them for regular walks, but don't overdo it, and remember that an older dog cannot handle the heat or cold as well as a young dog.

There is no good place to add the following discussion, so I might as well put it here. Keep in mind that there will come a time when an older dog may be suffering more than living. I like to let the dog tell me when it is time however. Generally speaking, a dog that can get around, is responsive and eating well is not ready to go. If they are not responsive, not eating well or not walking, the time may have come to make a difficult decision. Like so many things in this life, the difficult decisions are usually the right decisions. I know it is hard to part with a loyal friend, but if we keep a suffering pet alive with no chance of relieving their suffering, we are being selfish. Your veterinarian may help you make this decision, but only you can make the final decision. In many cases in my career it appears that euthanasia of a suffering animal has been a gift rather than a theft. The actual procedure involves an overdose of a barbiturate which is much like taking too many sleeping pills, and it is considered to be a peaceful way to go.

Paddling of the Feet

Paddling is usually associated with seizure type activity in the brain. It may be caused by a viral disease like distemper, a toxin like strychnine, or a metabolic problem like hypocalcemia. Sometimes it will also be seen in a dog while it is dreaming! One should seek veterinary help, especially if this sign is accompanied by others.

Paleness (Gums or Mucous Membranes)

This refers to paleness of the gums or mucous membranes, not the color of the fur. If a dog has white gums, or white conjunctiva (the tissue around the eyes,) it is probably anemic. This is an emergency and the dog should be seen by a veterinarian right away. **Fig. 37**

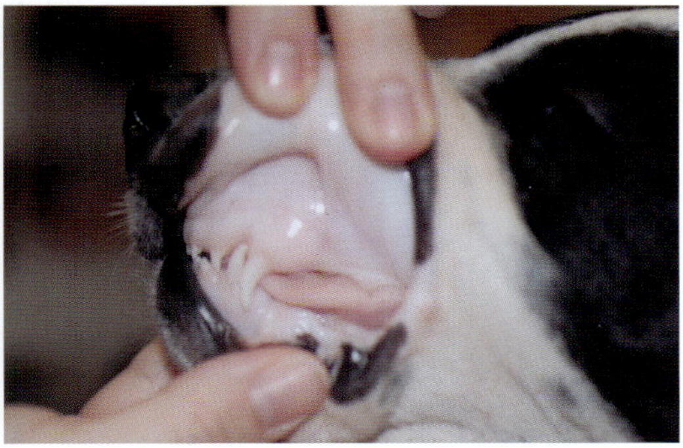

Fig. 37. Pale gums. This is a serious sign that often indicates either anemia or a major circulatory problem. See a veterinarian immediately.

Causes for anemia include fleas, ticks, worms, blood parasites, cancer, splenic rupture, or autoimmune hemolytic anemia(an unusual disease whereby the immune system begins attacking its own red blood cells).

If you suspect that fleas and worms are involved, and this is very likely with a puppy, you may attempt treatment at home. This will involve eliminating these parasites using some of the great products presently available. See the sections on fleas and worms and the drug chart for the names and doses of these products. An iron supplement may be helpful as well. Consult your veterinarian for the product they recommend. We use a product called Lixotinic® at the dose recommended in the drug chart.

In an older dog, professional help should be sought immediately, since there are more likely to be more serious and complicated causes involved.

Paralysis

The sudden loss of the ability to move either part or all of the body is a very frightening and life threatening situation. The usual cause is trauma to the head or spinal cord in the neck. In many other cases known or unknown toxins may be at work (e.g. botulism or the toxins produced by some ticks). In rare cases, an autoimmune disease may be at work or there may be a defect in the neuromuscular receptors (e.g. myasthenia gravis). Sudden paralysis of the rear legs may be due to the rupture of an intervertebral disc, putting pressure on the spinal cord. These diseases can not be diagnosed or treated at home. Transport your dog to the veterinarian right away. Remain calm. Many of these cases can and will respond to treatment.

Use a board or blanket to pick up such a dog. Be careful not to put any pressure on the head or neck. Consider the use of a muzzle since some dogs may still be able to move their heads and could bite out of fear or pain.

A history of trauma such as a fall, being hit by a car or a fight with a larger dog may be the cause of paralysis. Unless the spinal cord is severed, many of these injuries will respond to time and TLC (tender loving care). A veterinarian will often administer antibiotics for infections from bites or steroids and diuretics to reduce swelling of the spinal cord. Any wounds will need to be cleaned. During this recovery period, every need of the injured dog must be met. Sometimes a dog will require hand feeding or watering for days. They will also require cleaning if they soil themselves. Provide soft bedding during this time to prevent decubital ulcers (bed sores) from forming on the hips and shoulders. Keep in mind however that some injuries of this nature may result in permanent partial paralysis. Sometimes euthanasia should be considered. Consult with your veterinarian.

The gradual onset of paralysis and the presence of ticks on a dog suggest that you may be dealing with tick paralysis. It is believed that some ticks may produce a toxin resulting in a gradual total paralysis of a dog. Furthermore, it may only take one tick! Therefore, search your dog thoroughly for ticks and remove any that you find. Take care to use a pair of forceps or tweezers, not your fingers since you may expose yourself to several diseases by removing ticks with your bare hands. Flush the ticks and wash your hands afterwards. If ticks toxins are involved, the dog will gradually improve, once the tick is removed. Again, transport your dog to the veterinarian right away.

Pawing at the Eyes, Mouth, or Nose

Pawing at the eyes usually indicates a painful situation is present in the eyes. It may be a foreign object in the eye or severe inflammation secondary to an irritant or allergen. Sometimes, it because the eye is too dry. Flush the eye with water or saline and **see a veterinarian as soon as possible if there is no response. Fig. 38**

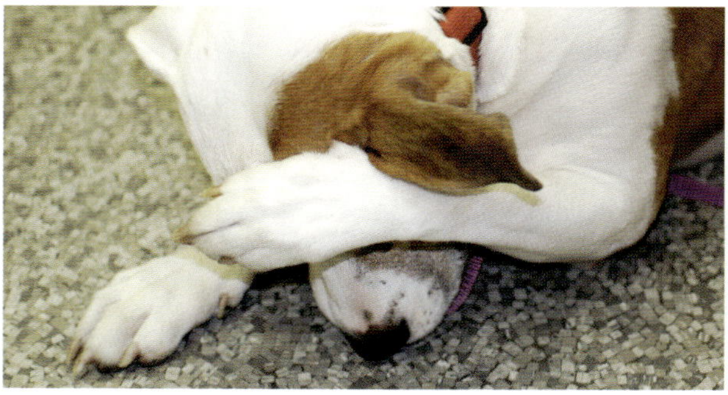

Fig. 38. Pawing at the eye. This sign suggests that there is a scratch in the surface of the eye, but may also be any irritating situation in that eye. One may attempt to flush out the eye with water or an eyewash solution.

In almost every case of pawing at the mouth (in dogs), a foreign object stuck between the teeth is involved. More often than not a stick or bone is stuck between the upper molars bridging the roof of the mouth. In some dogs, it may require sedation in order to remove the object, but sometimes the object can be seen and removed without sedation.

Sometimes there is a string wrapped around the teeth. Occasionally, a fish hook or some other sharp object is imbedded in the lip. These usually must be removed under general anesthesia.

In young dogs that are teething, the gums are usually inflamed and a dog may paw at the mouth even though there are no foreign objects present. Teething usually occurs between four and six months of age.

Pawing at the nose usually indicates that a foreign object is present in one of the nostrils. It may be accompanied by severe sneezing fits. If no object is visible that can be removed, **have your dog seen by a veterinarian right away.**

Penile or Vaginal Problems

A small amount of yellow discharge from the penis is considered normal for dogs and it is called smegma. A large amount of foul smelling discharge, particularly if there is any blood in it, is not normal. This probably is an infection of the preputial area, which may be either bacterial or viral. Antibiotics are suggested. **See your veterinarian**.

Rarely, the opening of the prepuce is too narrow for the penis. Thus, the penis can either not be extended, or it may get stuck if it does come out. A narrow opening may interfere with urination. If one notices that the penis is extended for any length of time, you should try to lubricate it with a sterile lubricant such as KY Jelly® and return it back inside the sheath. Sometimes you may have to pull the foreskin back and roll it outward, since hair may be trapped inside. **If you can not replace the penis back into its sheath, it may become more swollen. This is an emergency. Get that dog to a veterinarian right away.**

Vaginal swelling is normal during the time of estrus. However, continued swelling past the normal amount of time, or swelling at other times, along with a discharge may suggest that vaginitis is present.

A large amount of discharge along with a loss of appetite, and increased drinking could suggest an infection in the uterus called pyometra. This literally means that the uterus is full of pus! This is usually a surgical emergency, although antibiotics may be administered initially. **You must get your dog**

to the veterinarian right away. Keep in mind that in some cases of pyometra, there will be no discharge at all. The abdomen may feel full and "dough like" however.

Any tissue protruding from the vagina is not normal. The inside of the vagina may become so swollen that it protrudes. **Keep the tissue moist and get your dog to the veterinarian right away. This is an emergency!**

Poisoning

Poisoning occurs all too commonly in dogs. Prevention is the best treatment and this means dog-proofing your house and not leaving potential poisons out in the open. The most common poisonings occur from houseplants, rat or mouse poisons and antifreeze. Household cleansers, insecticides, and human medications or certain foods are also commonly involved.

Common indoor plants include Aloe, Corn Plants, Dieffenbachia, Pothos, Kalanchoe, Dracaena, Philodendrons, Ferns and others. Certain common outdoor plants are also deadly if consumed. These plants include Azaleas, Mountain Laurels, Oleanders, Lantana, Elephant Ears, Lilies, English Ivy, Bird of Paradise, Yew, Ferns, and many vines. Sago Palms are very dangerous and a number of true palms produce very toxic seeds.

Mouse or rat poisons usually contain anticoagulants called coumarins that cause internal bleeding. While they are not painful, they are generally deadly to dogs of all sizes. Small dogs are particularly susceptible since they are more likely to consume a lethal dose.

Antifreeze products containing ethylene glycol are sweet and readily consumed by dogs. It doesn't take much to result in fatal kidney damage.

Household cleansers and detergents are very dangerous if consumed. Other products to watch for are fabric softeners, solvents, bleach, lighter fluid, drain cleaners and oven sprays. Most insecticides are extremely toxic as well.

Human medications that can be especially dangerous include ibuprofen, acetaminophen, prednisone, anticancer medications, antidepressants, tranquilizers, anti-seizure medications, many antihistamines and other cold and flu medications

Foods that we would never expect to be toxic to dogs but are very dangerous include chocolate, onions, and avocados. Even grapes and raisins have been associated with irreversible and fatal kidney damage in dogs! The cause is still unknown. Coffee has also been known to be toxic in large quantities.

THE BEST THING TO DO IN CASES OF POISONING IS TO GET YOUR DOG TO THE VETERINARIAN RIGHT AWAY! BRING THE POISONOUS PRODUCT, CONTAINER, OR PLANT WITH YOU!

IF THE POISON WAS JUST INGESTED (WITHIN 30 – 60 MINUTES) AND IT IS A NON-CORROSIVE AGENT (SEE THE LABEL), VOMITING SHOULD BE INDUCED WITH HYDROGEN PEROXIDE. ONE TO FIVE TABLESPOONS SHOULD BE GIVEN DEPENDING UPON THE SIZE OF THE DOG. VOMITING WILL OFTEN OCCUR WITHIN 15 MINUTES. IF NO VOMITING OCCURS, REPEAT THE PROCESS. THE LABEL OF THE PRODUCT CONSUMED WILL OFTEN ADVISE IF VOMITING SHOULD BE INDUCED OR NOT. HOWEVER, IF IN DOUBT, GET IT OUT! The damage to the upper GI tract if vomiting is induced is usually far less severe that the damage that might be done if the product gets absorbed, in terms of liver and kidney disease. ***See the veterinary poison advice numbers listed in the appendices on page 78 if in doubt.***

The veterinarian may then follow up with the administration of an antidote, supportive care and probably blood work to determine the extent of the damage done. A slurry of activated charcoal may be given. Gastrointestinal protectants such as Kaopectate®, Pepto Bismol® or Carafate® may be dispensed. Follow their recommendations. It may save your dog's life.

Puppy Problems (Pediatrics)

Puppies are prone to a variety of problems. These include low body temperature (hypothermia), low blood sugar (hypoglycemia), and dehydration, which are potential problems common to all neonatal mammals. Small breed dogs may also be a risk for low blood calcium (hypocalcemia). **Fig. 39**

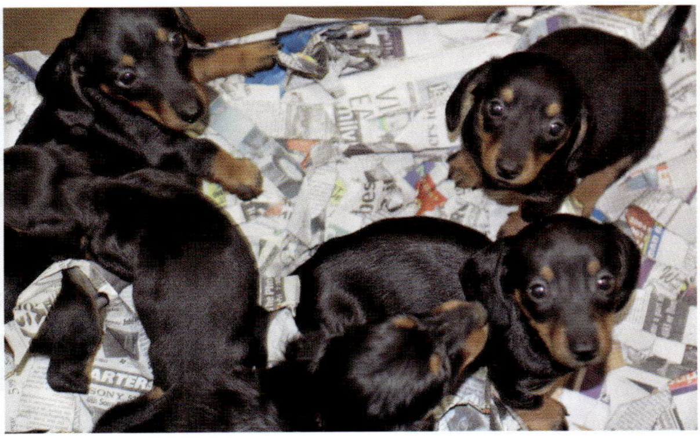

Fig. 39. Puppies. They are very cute but come with a lot of responsibility. Get them vaccinated properly and puppy proof your house. Feed them an appropriate diet.

One of the leading causes of death for young puppies is suffocation, as they may get trapped under the mother at times. You will improve survival of the puppies by providing them with some traction so they can crawl away from the mother if she rolls over. The best way to do this is to provide some indoor/outdoor carpet as the substrate for the mother and puppies. It is easy to clean, easy to replace and gives the puppies good traction.

If puppies are being fostered, there is a risk that they will aspirate the milk replacer that they are being given. Avoid this by feeding them small amounts at a time and holding the puppies in a vertical, rather than horizontal position while you are feeding them. Also, do not make the hole in the nipple too big. If the puppy aspirates, they may gag, cough and spit up milk or blow some out the nose. The breathing may become rapid and sound moist. If this occurs, turn the puppy upside down and see if anything runs out of the mouth. This is both helpful and diagnostic for aspiration. You may want to seek professional help if this occurs, as milk in the lungs may result in a respiratory infection.

The opposite of taking in too much milk replacer is not drinking at all. Very weak, cold and dehydrated puppies may not nurse or suckle voluntarily. In this case, tube feeding is the treatment of choice. A soft rubber tube with a rounded end, such as a stomach tube or a French catheter can be gently inserted into the puppies stomach and a meal delivered. One may first place the tube on the outside of the puppy and mark a distance on the tube that spans from the mouth to the last rib. This will mark the distance to the stomach so that the tube may be inserted the appropriate distance. Mix the powdered milk fresh each time and administer it to the puppy. Do not use old formula. When placing the tube, make sure the puppy's neck is not straight, and that the puppy is not on its back. Administer the formula slowly. Overfeeding or feeding a mixture that is too rich often results in diarrhea. Underfeeding is usually recognized by a constantly crying puppy. **Use a commercial milk replacer not cow's milk. A substitute formula that can be used until a commercial milk replacer can be purchased has been recommended in the *Dog Owner's Home Veterinary Handbook*. It is 8 oz of whole milk, 3 egg yolks, 1 tablespoon of corn oil, and one drop of liquid pediatric vitamins. Usually, a newborn puppy will consume ½ to 1 tsp. of formula for its first several meals, but weigh that puppy and follow the instructions on the can of milk replacer.**

Young puppies have very little protection against the serious viral diseases of dogs. While they receive protection in the form of maternal antibodies, it is often not sufficient to protect them entirely from these diseases. Diseases such as canine distemper and parvo are fatal for many puppies. If the mother dog is vaccinated regularly, it will provide the puppy with better protection. Also the overall health of the puppies will help to determine their resistance, so worms must be eliminated by a regular deworming protocol. I recommend a deworming every 2 weeks starting as early as 2 weeks of age with pyrantel pamoate (Strongid T®) at a dose of 1 ml/10 pounds of body weight. *See the section on worms*.

Diarrhea is a common and very serious problem in puppies. Sometimes it is a transient problem due to something as simple as milk replacer that is too rich. Sometimes it may be due to toxic milk from the mother. Sometimes it may be due to parasites. The worst case scenario though, is an infection with a viral disease such as parvo or corona virus. Such an infection will probably require professional help if the puppy is to have a chance to survive. IV fluids and antibiotics among other things will be required. **Home management of short-term diarrhea in a puppy includes oral fluid replacement. Pedialyte® works excellently. See the section on dehydration for determining the amount to give. GI protectants are also very helpful.**

The sudden onset of vomiting in a puppy is a serious sign. It usually suggests that the puppy has ingested a foreign object. Parts of toys, small items of clothing (like socks or stockings), and especially string may all become deadly if not removed. Other things which may cause vomiting include toxicity from spoiled foods, intestinal worms, and a rare situation in which the intestine folds over on itself like a sock. This is called an intussusception. Aggressive veterinary care and even surgery may be required if one of these events occurs. **If the puppy appears bright and alert, and is not dehydrated, not febrile(feverish), and doesn't have concurrent diarrhea (especially bloody diarrhea) with the vomiting, one may attempt to pass a suspected small foreign object by administering a bulk laxative such as Metamucil® every four hours for two days at a dose similar to that for a child.** *See the drug chart*. However, if the vomiting persists and no foreign object is observed in the stool during that time, veterinary care should be sought. The veterinarian will be likely to recommend radiographs (X-rays) and may even advise surgery. If the radiographs don't show an obvious foreign object, and the puppy is stable, my "magic number" for considering surgery is about 5 days for most dogs, but it varies with size and condition. This is especially true if the puppy is capable of keeping down fluids, and maybe even a small amount of food. See the section on vomiting for a further discussion of vomiting.

If a puppy's eyes are swollen and there is some pus leaking from one corner, this is likely to be an infection called neonatal opthalmitis. The eyelids must be teased open to allow the pus to drain. A topical ophthalmic antibiotic may then be placed in each eye. *See the section on eye problems* and consider seeking professional help in order to reduce the risk of permanent damage. **See Fig. 16.**

A nasal discharge, gasping, sneezing, wheezing, or coughing all suggest that there may be a respiratory infection or some other respiratory system problem. Aspiration of formula may have occurred. This is very serious. Get that puppy to a veterinarian right away. Antibiotics may be necessary. Sometimes nebulization with bronchodilators or other agents may be useful. Occasionally respiratory problems in a puppy are secondary to a congenital defect such as a cleft palate or heart defect. Again, this usually requires a veterinarian to diagnose and possibly treat.

A sudden seizure in a young puppy is most likely due to low blood sugar (hypoglycemia.) This is most common in small breed puppies. *See the section below on seizures and shaking*.

Scooting

Scooting is a term applied to a dog that is rubbing its rear end (usually the anal area) on the floor or ground. There are generally three reasons that this occurs. The most common reason is intestinal worms. The second most common reason is that the anal glands are full. The third most common reason is fleas, and possibly an allergy to them. Treat for worms *(see the section on worms)*, express the anal glands if you know how(or have a groomer or veterinary technician do it) and treat for fleas. If that doesn't stop the problem, or if you notice any very firm lumps in the area of the anus, see your veterinarian.

Seizures and Shaking (Fits)

The two main causes for seizures in dogs are hypoglycemia and epilepsy, but there are many other possible causes. A seizure may be recognized by sudden collapse and extension of the legs. Sometimes breathing may temporarily stop. Then they may begin shaking. Sometimes it is associated with chewing motions and frothing at the mouth. Wild paddling of the legs may be observed. They may soil themselves.

Hypoglycemia is seen primarily in puppies and first aid for this involves the administration of oral glucose. Karo Syrup®, Coca Cola®, or even better, crushed glucose tablets will work very well. Usually, small breed puppies are more commonly affected. Sometimes this will be insufficient to stop a seizure, and a veterinarian may have to administer IV glucose. Keep the puppy warm and rush it to a veterinarian right away.

Epilepsy is the presence of abnormal electrical impulses in the brain. It results in seizures that may be quite severe or very mild. These seizures may also vary in frequency; some dogs have seizures daily, while others have them once or twice a year! Both the severity and frequency of the seizures will determine if a dog needs treatment. Mild, infrequent seizures will rarely be treated by a veterinarian, but severe or frequent seizures will require treatment.

Another cause for seizures and shaking is hypocalcemia, which is also known as eclampsia. This is most commonly seen in small breed female dogs which have just delivered puppies. See the discussion on collapse.

A seizure is a scary thing to observe, but keep in mind that they are usually not life threatening. **Stay calm, and provide padding around the dog if necessary to prevent them from injuring themselves. If the seizure is occurring in a dangerous location, such as near sharp objects or in a street, attempt to move the dog to a safer location. Otherwise do not disturb the affected dog as this may worsen the seizure or start a new one. Seek professional help immediately if the seizure continues for more than five minutes. Do not put your hand in the dog's mouth for any purpose. If they are biting their tongue, try to insert a towel or other soft object between the teeth to cushion the bite. However, this is not common, and dogs can not swallow their tongues, so the best thing is often to leave them alone.**

If you have any Diazepam (Valium®) tablets you may crush the tablet and mix it with some water in a syringe and administer it rectally. Some of the diazepam may be absorbed this way and this may lessen the severity of the seizure while the dog is being transported to the veterinarian.

A unique kind of mild seizure involves what is called a "chewing gum seizure". This seizure receives its name because the affected dog may begin a repetitive "chewing" motion. The most likely cause for this is damage to the brain caused by the distemper virus. Another less common cause for this unusual sign is heavy metal poisoning e.g. lead toxicity. **Have your dog seen by your veterinarian right away**. They may recommend some blood work to determine a possible cause.

Tremors may be considered minor seizures in many cases. Seek professional help immediately to determine the cause and prescribe the treatment.

Shaking the Head

A dog usually shakes its head if there is an ear problem. Usually, ear mites or an ear infection is to blame. However, there may be a foreign object in the ear, including fleas, ticks, or perhaps something more ominous, such as a small tumor. Vigorous side to side shaking may result in ruptured blood vessels in the ears. They may look like little water filled balloons. However, they are filled with blood, and left untreated, these blood clots will contract and deform the ears. Veterinarians refer to these blood pockets in the ears as hematomas, and they should be called upon to treat them.

Another reason for head shaking is a cut at the tip of the ear. This can be due to a bite or any other trauma. It may itch the dog and they may shake their heads violently. If the tip of the ear is bleeding, it may result in a bloody mess as drops of blood are spattered everywhere. Perhaps the best treatment under these circumstances is to apply a piece of gauze to the tip of the ear and bandage it to the top of the head with a broad bandage wrapped behind the other ear and completely around the neck. This should stop or slow the bleeding until a veterinarian can be seen. **Fig. 40, Fig. 41**

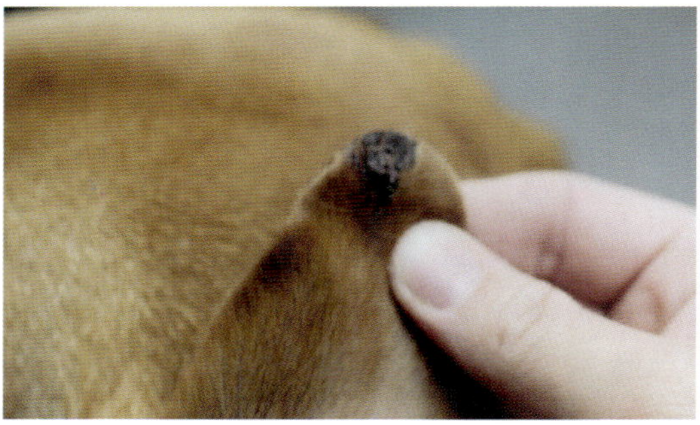

Fig. 40. Lesion at tip of ear. Cuts at the tip of the ear will often result in a bloody mess as the dogs sling their ears. A variety of causes are possible, including trauma and fly bites, but always check inside the ear for evidence of infection. See the next fig...

Fig. 41. Ear bandaged to top of head. Bandaging an ear over the top of the head is the best first aid for a bleeding ear. Apply gauze to the bleeding area and then flatten the ear against the top of the head with a broad medical tape. The tape may then be wrapped around the neck behind the other ear, encircling the entire neck.

See the section on ear problems.

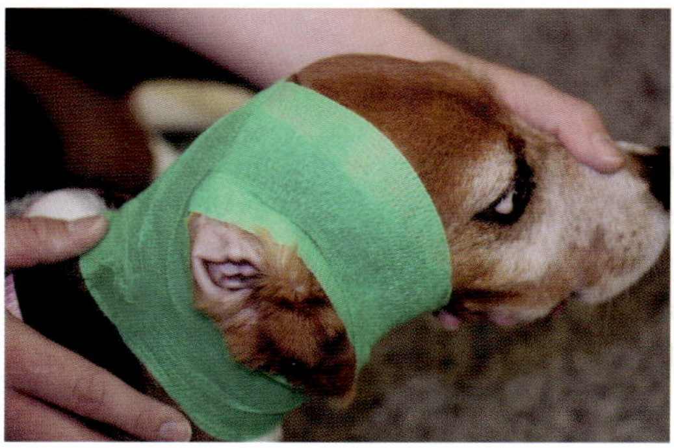

Sneezing (and Nasal Discharge)

Sneezing by itself is not usually a serious sign in a dog although it can be a precursor of things to come which may be worse. It can be one of the early signs of a respiratory infection, including infectious tracheobronchitis or distemper. It is most likely to be caused by an allergy to something in the environment, such as a carpet cleaner or detergent. Dust, dander from other animals, house dust mites, molds and a plethora of other things may cause an allergic reaction, such as sneezing, itchiness, or runny eyes.

If an allergy is suspected, one may try using an unscented cleanser. One common reason for increased sneezing is cigarette smoke. So if you are smoking around your dog and it is sneezing frequently, try to take a break and see if the sneezing subsides.

One other possibility for sneezing is sinusitis, an inflammation of the sinuses. This may be infectious in nature, and a dental infection may be at the root of the problem (no pun intended). In a small dog, an infection near the roots of the teeth can easily erode through the thin bone and into the sinuses. If sneezing occurs concurrently with obvious signs of dental disease (tartar, discoloration of the teeth, or redness of the gums,) **seek veterinary care immediately.**

Chronic sinusitis may also be due to a fungal infection, a foreign object in the nose or even a nasal tumor. None of these can be diagnosed or treated at home so one should seek veterinary attention whenever chronic sneezing is observed.

Nasal discharges often accompany sneezing but not always. Sometimes they occur without sneezing. The causes are similar however. Interestingly, the nature of the discharge will often give a clue as to the cause. A clear discharge usually indicates an allergic reaction, while a colored discharge (green or yellow) usually indicates an infection.

Any nose bleeds should be considered serious and require immediate veterinary attention. Several diseases including erlichiosis, anaplasmosis, or rickettsiosis may be the cause, but any chronic sinusitis may eventually become severe enough to bleed. Bleeding from the nose may also be seen when rat poison has been ingested, most of which contain anticoagulants. **Immediate attention is required since internal bleeding or bleeding from another orifice may be imminent if a rodenticide has been consumed.** *See Fig. 5.*

Staggering

See the discussion on dizziness. Toxins are usually to blame for sudden onsets of staggering. These could include bacterial toxins, or those from chemicals or heavy metals. Toads and many plants (including marijuana) also contain toxins capable of causing staggering. Spider or snake bites are also capable of delivering venom that can result in staggering. Many of these toxins will be associated with other signs such as vomiting, diarrhea or swelling somewhere. Sometimes staggering occurs following a seizure or a stroke. Trauma to the head may also result in the sudden onset of staggering. Furthermore, there are a large number of inherited neuropathies (nerve disorders) and myopathies (muscle disorders) that may affect dogs.

This is a serious sign that cannot be diagnosed or treated at home. Get that dog to a veterinarian right away. The only first aid treatment that can be administered at home is to rinse out the mouth repeatedly with a garden hose if the dog has just mouthed a toad or other toxic substance.

Swallowing Problems

Difficult swallowing is usually associated with an inflammation of the throat. The most common reason is the ingestion of some irritating substance or toxic plant. It may also be due to an infection of the throat or tonsils. Another reason this may occur is if there is a partial blockage of the esophagus, the tube leading to the stomach. Rarely, the muscle of the esophagus may become atonic and it may stretch. This is referred to as megaesophagus. There may be an autoimmune component to this disorder. A sudden onset of difficulty swallowing suggests the ingestion of a foreign object or irritant (plant or chemical), while a slow onset suggests an infectious process or a tumor. Puppies that suddenly develop this problem are likely to have ingested a foreign object, while those that develop it slowly may have a neurological problem that they were born with. None of these things can be diagnosed at home. **Get that puppy or dog to a veterinarian right away.** Difficult swallowing may be associated with regurgitation as well. *See the discussion on vomiting and regurgitation.*

Swelling of Any Surface or Appendage

Swelling of any surface is abnormal in dogs. Swelling around the face may indicate a dental abscess, swelling of the abdomen often indicates that there is fluid in the abdomen, swelling in the armpits or behind the knees may indicate a tumor of the lymph nodes and swelling of the joints suggests inflammation or an infection of the joint. Every one of these problems must be evaluated by a veterinarian. Furthermore, there are other causes for the signs described above; those listed are just the most common. **Fig. 42**

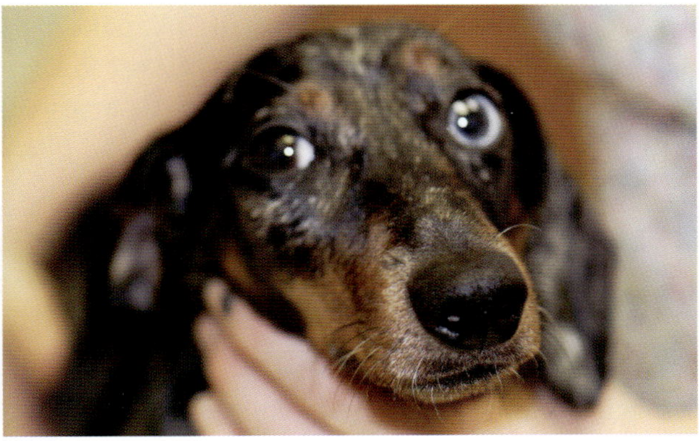

Fig. 42. Swelling below right eye. Often, the cause for this is an abscessed carnassial tooth (the largest molar in the upper jaw right below the eye). It may need to be removed, which is no easy task.

Another area that may be swollen is an arm or leg. This suggests either trauma to that appendage, with a possible fracture, or an infection. If a dog is still using a swollen leg, it is more likely to be an infection rather than a fracture. Antibiotics may be tried if one has access to them, especially if there is evidence of a bite i.e. Puncture wounds. Warm compresses placed on the swollen area for five minutes twice daily may also be effective. However, if the cause of the swelling is a fractured leg or a circulatory problem, these methods will not work. You must seek the help of a veterinarian. See the discussion on dragging a leg, carrying a leg or limping.

A swollen toe is likely to be a fractured toe, but usually it is not necessary to attempt to splint one toe as the other toes generally stabilize it enough to allow healing. There are exceptions however.

A swollen face is usually due to an acute allergic reaction to an insect, spider, or snake bite. An allergic reaction may also have been caused by exposure to an irritating plant or some chemical irritant in the environment or home. Sometimes, the face may be swollen on one side right below the eye. This may be due to an abscess of the largest molar in the upper jaw. If the swelling shows up rapidly, consider using diphenhydramine at the dose listed in the drug chart, since this is likely to be an allergic reaction. If the swelling shows up primarily on one side, a molar abscess is more likely.

Swelling of the genital area in either males or females suggests either an infection or trauma. **Seek veterinary help immediately.** S*ee the section on penile or vaginal problems*.

Trauma

A fall, a deep scratch, a fight, or a run in with a car all qualify as traumatic events. A dog may become shocky, the heart rate will be rapid, but the circulation is compromised. Limbs will feel cold, and the gums will look pale. This is an emergency! **Get that dog to a veterinarian right away.** Cover to keep warm, apply pressure to stop any bleeding, and transport as soon as possible. *See elsewhere in this book for first aid for specific signs of trauma i.e. bites, bleeding, first aid for miscellaneous problems, collapse, etc.*

Torn Nails and Torn Pads

Sudden limping and pain with bleeding may be associated with a torn nail. Typically a nail is coming out at an unusual angle and it may be bleeding, sometimes profusely. The reason for this is usually a nail that has been torn at the base. This is very painful, and dogs will often limp or scream in pain if the nail is touched. It is often best to have the dog sedated and the have the entire nail removed. Unless bleeding is severe, no emergency treatment is required. However, if there is a lot of bleeding, one may attempt to stop it by applying a cyanoacrylate glue to the base of the broken nail without moving the nail. While this may burn some, the pain will often be very brief. **Get that dog to a veterinarian**, who will remove the nail under sedation, as mentioned above. **Fig. 43**

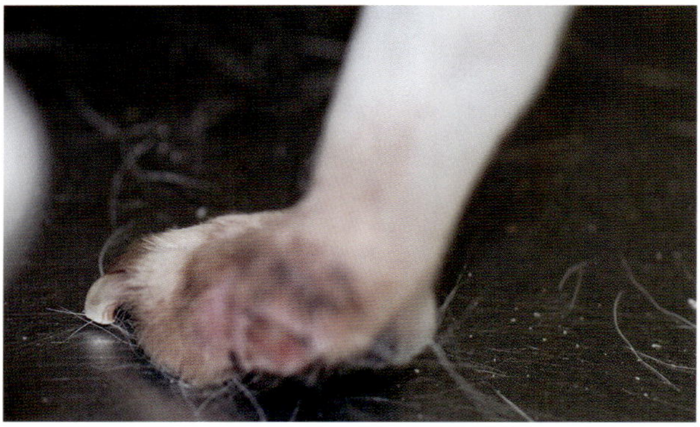

Fig. 43. Torn nail. A torn nail and exposed nail bed is painful for the dog and may be bleeding. Many kinds of powder, like flour or corn-starch may stop the bleeding, but the nail may have to be removed. Unless it is very loose and your dog is very cooperative, this may require sedation.

A torn pad is painful for the dog but not usually an emergency. Depending upon the size of the piece that is torn, and how well it is attached, it may be snipped off with a sharp scissor. A tiny piece may be removed quickly. A larger piece however, may require sedation in order to remove. If you are not sure, check with your veterinarian. The open area will granulate in (fill in with tissue) in several days or weeks. Sometimes a bandage may be required but this is rare. Most of the time, just keeping the affected dog on a clean, carpetless floor for several days will work once the loose piece of pad is removed.

Urination Problems

If a dog is urinating very frequently, or straining to urinate, or has any blood in its urine, it has a problem.

Frequent urination may be caused by a simple urinary tract infection, the presence of bladder or kidney stones, kidney disease, diabetes insipidus, diabetes mellitus or rarely, a tumor of the bladder. In male dogs, prostate problems also may be present. In older female dogs, hypoestrogenism may lead to incontinence as well. However, it may simply be associated with increased water consumption, which may occur for a variety of reasons. Some dogs just like to drink a lot! None of these problems may be diagnosed at home, so the owner is advised to seek veterinary help immediately.

Blood in the urine suggests that an infection or stones are present, while normal appearing urine may suggest that a metabolic problem such as diabetes mellitus (too much sugar in the blood and urine) or diabetes insipidus (there is no control over the concentration of the urine) is the likely cause.

Dribbling urine at night often suggests a possible prostate problem in a male dog or hypoestrogenism (very low estrogen level) in female dogs. The typical history is that of a male dog (unneutered) that is dribbling between urinations or a spayed (neutered) female dog that is dribbling at night while she sleeps. For a male dog the most likely prostate problem is benign prostatic hypertrophy (BPH), and this usually responds to neutering plus antibiotic for a short time. For a female dog, treatment involves supplementation with estrogen. We usually use DES (diethyl stilbesterol) at a dose of 1 mg per day for three days then 1 mg per week for 7 weeks. But there are many other possibilities for dribbling.

Straining to urinate is often seen with bladder stones. A complete blockage may occur if a small stone blocks the urethra. **Fig. 44**

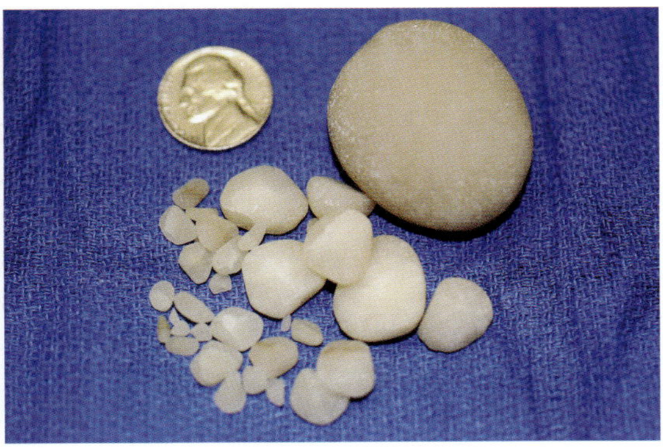

Fig. 44. Bladder stones. These stones were removed from one dog's bladder. Many stones can be dissolved by using the proper diet, but different kinds of stones require different foods, and some kinds of stones will not respond well to dietary management. Thus they may need to be removed surgically.

Hence, urination difficulties need to be addressed by a veterinarian as soon as possible. Home remedies during the interim may include encouraging increased fluid consumption, including those that are acidic in most cases. These would include things like cranberry juice, blackberry juice and the citrus juices(even though these are often not very palatable to most dogs). However, water is the best home medicine in this case. Give water, and lots of it!

In many cases of stone formation, diet is to blame. Typically, diets that are high in mineral content (referred to as ash content in many veterinary references) contribute to this problem. Dairy products, such as milk and cheese, are not suitable snacks for many dogs, since they contain high levels of minerals, especially those dogs suffering from urinary tract problems.

Vocalization

Dogs bark for a number of reasons including excitement, fear, hostility or some need. They may be hungry, thirsty, or need to go outside to defecate or urinate. They may be trying to communicate something else to you. Sometimes they may just be bored and want to go for a walk.

In some cases, they may whine or cry out in pain. These vocalizations may be sudden or prolonged over a period of time. A sudden, loud repetitious cry or scream indicates severe pain, and the dog should be taken to a veterinarian right away. If a dog is screaming and has a severe injury suggesting that it may be in pain, be careful when approaching and attempting to move it. It may bite out of pain or fear. Some have suggested using a belt as a muzzle prior to attempting to move a large dog. A large towel may be thrown over a small dog prior to picking it up.

Screaming during sleep may indicate a bad dream. It is often associated with some movement, such as paddling of the legs.

Excessive or constant barking is usually a behavioral rather than medical problem. Boredom or the need for some attention is often to blame. You may wish to consult a trainer or behaviorist if the problem persists.

Vomiting (and Regurgitation)

Vomiting is a common problem seen in dogs. It is not always an emergency, particularly if it only happens once or twice. However, if the vomiting is persistent, or if accompanied by anorexia and diarrhea, s**eek veterinary help immediately.** The causes for vomiting are numerous. Most of the time it is likely to be what veterinarians call "acute dietary indiscretion." which is a fancy way of saying that the patient ate something that he or she shouldn't have! First aid treatment for such an act usually involves two things, and they can be easily accomplished at home. **Fig. 45**

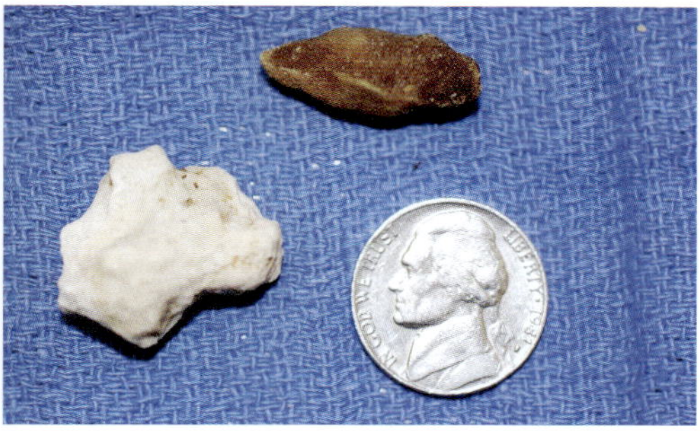

Fig. 45. Ingested stones. Puppies will swallow just about anything. These stones were passed by a puppy after several days of receiving metamucil® laxative.

Firstly, don't feed your dog for 12 to 24 hours. Rest that gut! This is the best thing you can do in many cases. Many dogs may not want to eat during this time anyway.

Secondly, one may administer a gastrointestinal protectant such as Kaopectate® or Peptobismol® at the dose listed in the drug chart. Antacid agents such as Pepcid®, Tagamet®, or Zantac® can also be administered at the dose recommended in the drug chart. Sometimes a bulk laxative like Metamucil® at the dose recommended in the drug chart is helpful at passing some foreign objects.

Thirdly, when starting to feed again, feed something bland, like baked, skinless, white meat chicken and rice. One may also use a bland food designed for this purpose called Hill's Prescription Diet I/D®. Feed a small amount (a few tablespoons.) Wait an hour and if no vomiting occurs, offer another small meal of similar size. Repeat the process several more times and then offer a small quantity of the regular dog food after 6 – 12 hours. If no vomiting occurs then, consider the problem solved.

Persistent vomiting is a different story. There are many causes and some of these are extremely serious. Viral infections, including parvo and corona, as well as intestinal parasites, foreign objects, ulcers, tumors, kidney disease, liver disease, pancreatitis and many other things may cause vomiting. None of these can be diagnosed at home, so a dog that is vomiting persistently should be seen by a veterinarian as soon as possible.

Regurgitation differs from vomiting in that it is a non-forceful expulsion of undigested food. A dog may eat, but several minutes to hours later, the undigested food may come back up. The most common reason this happens suddenly is that a foreign object is stuck in the esophagus. There are a number of other reasons that this problem may occur but none of these can be diagnosed or treated at home. Get your dog to a veterinarian right away or he/she may slowly starve. First aid may include feeding small, soft meals from an elevated position.

Worms (Intestinal)

If you have had a dog for any length of time, you will eventually see worms appear in the anal area or in the stool. Worms are parasites which rob dogs of energy and nutrients. They may cause vomiting and diarrhea and could increase the likelihood of a secondary bacterial or viral infection. If left untreated, they will often kill their host. **Fig. 46**

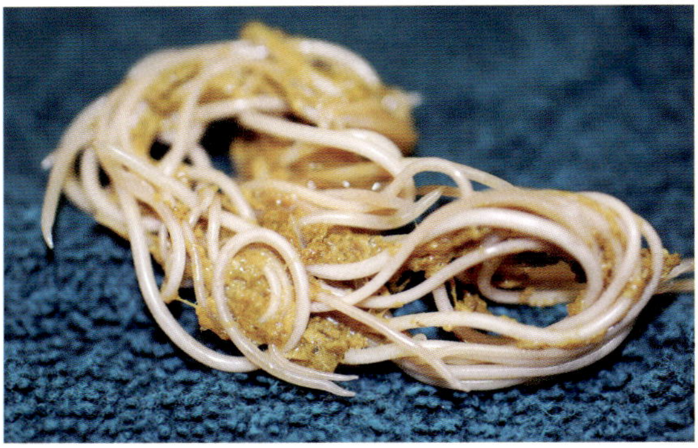

Fig. 46. Worms. Worms are not usually this obvious in the stool of affected dogs. Many times dogs just pass their eggs, which are microscopic. Have a fecal exam (microscopic examination of the feces) performed at least once per year.

In adult dogs, the worm you are most likely to encounter is the tapeworm *Dipylidium caninum*. Tapeworms may be recognized most frequently as "grain of rice" sized segments on the stool. Initially, they are white and may be observed elongating and contracting. They will appear flat if one examines them closely. Later, these segments will dry out and truly do look like uncooked grains of rice. These segments contain the eggs. The life cycle of this species of worm is very interesting and involves the flea. Fleas ingest the dried segments and serve as the intermediate host for this worm. When an infected flea is swallowed, the dog gets tapeworms. Thus, any attempt to eliminate tapeworms must be tied to an effort to eliminate fleas. See the section on flea control. Other species of tapeworm exist, but this is the most common species. All species though may be eliminated using a drug called praziquantel at the dose recommended in the drug chart. This drug is usually only available from a veterinarian, either by injection or in a pill form. We recommend that the dose be repeated two weeks after the intial dose. Over the counter medications exist for the treatment of tapeworms, but they are not generally as safe or effective as this drug. This is not to say that tapeworms are the only worms that adult dogs get, but this is the most common species. They are susceptible to all of the worms listed in this section.

In puppies, the worm you are most likely to encounter is the roundworm. They appear long, round in cross section, and pointed on each end. A heavily infected puppy may have such a heavy load that the abdomen is very distended.

Sometimes, they will pass one or more of these worms in the stool, but this is not always the case and any puppy with a distended abdomen should be suspected of having roundworms, and possibly other species as well. Over the counter treatment may be successfully a accomplished by using a drug called pyrantel pamoate (Evict®, Strongid T®) at the dose recommended in the drug chart. A puppy so treated may pass a huge number of worms that looks like a pile of spaghetti! *See Fig. 46*

Perhaps the deadliest of the common worms are hookworms. These worms literally hook into the lining of the intestinal tract and drink blood. They will rapidly drain the blood, energy and life from a dog. Unfortunately, these worms are rarely seen or recognized if they are seen in the stool. But their presence is often readily recognized. The most common sign is dark stools. The darkness is due to the presence of digested blood! The consistency varies from solid, to tarry, to very loose and watery diarrhea, but the color is almost always dark. These worms will also be killed by the administration of pyrantel pamoate, as listed above for roundworms at the dose listed in the drug chart. We also use ivermectin injections to eliminate hookworms once we ascertain that a dog is heartworm negative. An injection of ivermectin has an advantage over pyrantel pamoate in some cases since it cannot be vomited. But if it is used in a dog with heartworms it may result in sudden death, so only veterinarians should administer ivermectin once the heartworm status of the dog is known. The dose for ivermectin is found in the drug chart. ***WARNING: NEVER USE IVERMECTIN IN THIS MANNER WITH COLLIES, SHELTIES, OR MIXES WITH THESE BREEDS. THEY ARE VERY SENSITIVE TO IVERMECTIN.***

The last common species of worm seen in dogs is the whipworm. So named because they are large on one end and small on the other, these worms usually live in the large intestine and cause enough irritation to result in chronic diarrhea. However, the history of the diarrhea is unusual in that it is often intermittent, and sometimes mucousy. These worms are very difficult to diagnose, and are often not seen on single fecal exams. Repeated microscopic fecal exams should be performed on any dog showing intermittent mucous stools or diarrhea. These worms will not be eliminated by using pyrantel pamoate. We usually use a drug called fenbendazole (Panacur®) at a dose listed in the drug chart. Ivermectin may also be used if the precautions listed above are taken (i.e. Make sure that the dog is heartworm negative.)

Appendices

PROBLEM/SOLUTION CHART (MOST LIKELY CAUSES)

Problem	Probable Causes	First Treatment
Abdominal Swelling	Heart Disease, Tumor, Fat	See Vet
Anorexia	Dietary Indiscretion, Many others	GI Protectants
Bad Breath	Dental Disease, Poor Digestion	Brush Teeth, Vet
Behavioral Problems	Bad Experience, Medical Problem	Trainer or Vet
Bites	Dog Fight	Clean Wounds, Vet
Bleeding	Trauma, HBC, Bites, Rat Poison	Pressure, Vet
Breathing Problems	Heart Disease, Respiratory Infection	Keep Cool, Vet
Collapse	Heart Disease, Hypoglycemia	Oral Glucose, Vet
Constipation	Diet, Age, Poor Colon Function	Bulk Laxative, Diet
Diarrhea	Dietary, Parasites, GI Virus	GI Protectants, Vet
Dizziness	Hypoglycemia, Neurological	Oral Glucose, Vet
Dragging Rear Legs	Spinal Trauma, IV Disc Disease	See Vet ASAP
Frothing at the Mouth	Tasted Something Toxic	Wash Mouth, Vet?
Hair Loss	Allergy (Fleas, Airborne, Food)	See Vet
Hunching Over	Abdominal Pain	See Vet ASAP
Itching	Allergy (Fleas, Airborne, Food)	See Vet
Lethargy	Anything	See Vet
Licking	Soreness, Stinging, Itching	See Vet
Lumps and Bumps	Tumor, Cyst, Hives, Infection	See Vet
Obesity	Dietary, Hypothyroidism	Diet, See Vet
Pale Gums	Anemia, Shock	See Vet ASAP
Protrusions(Prolapses)	Colon, penis, uterus,vagina	Lubricate and push back in. See Vet.
Seizures and Shaking	Epilepsy, Hypoglycemia, Others	See Vet ASAP
Shivering	Cold, Fever, Metabolic Problem	Warm, See Vet
Sneezing	Allergy, URI, Foreign Object in Nose	See Vet
Staggering	Toxin or Trauma, Neurological	See Vet
Swelling	Trauma, Infection	See Vet
Face	Bite (Snake, Insect), Abscessed Tooth	Benadryl,Vet
Legs	Bite (Dog, Snake), HBC, Heart Disease	See Vet
Trauma	HBC, Dog Bite	See Vet
Urination Problems	Infection, Diet,Prostate,Low Estrogen	See Vet
Vomiting (and Regurgitation)	Dietary, Foreign Body, Parasites	NPO, See Vet
Worms	From Mother, Soil, Fleas, Wild Foods	OTC Dewormer or See Vet

Abbreviations

ASAP	As Soon As Possible.
GI	Gastrointestinal (stomach or intestinal). Protectants include Kaopectate or Peptobismol
HBC	Hit By Car
IV	Intervertebral (between the bones of the spine)
NPO	No Food (usually 12 to 24 hours) to allow gut to rest
OTC	Over the Counter (not requiring a prescription)

Drugs Commonly Used in Dogs

Drug	Dose	Purpose
Advantage®	topically q 3 – 4 weeks	fleas
Advantix®	topically q 3 – 4 weeks	fleas and ticks
Amikacin	10 mg/kg IV,IM,SC	antibiotic
Aminophylline	10 mg/kg PO, IM, SC TID	bronchodilator
Amitrytiline(Elavil®)	2 mg/kg PO BID	anxiety,obsessive beh.
Amoxicillin	10-20mg/kg PO, BID	antibiotic
Aspirin	5 – 30 mg/kg PO, SID	antiinflammatory
Atopica®	5mg/kg SID x 14 days, wean off	allergy relief
Atropine	.02 – 1.5 mg/kg SC, IM, IV PRN	antidote
Azithromycin	10mg/kg PO, SID	antibiotic
Brewer's Yeast	200 mg/kg PO, SID	B vitamin suppl.
Butorphanol (Torbugesic®)	0.5- 1.0 mg/kg PO,SC,IM,IV q6-12h	analgesic
Carprofen (Rimadyl®)	2.2 mg/kg PO,SC, IV BID	analgesic
Cephalexin	22 mg/kg PO BID (standard)	antibiotic
Cimetidine (Tagamet®)	10 mg/kg PO, SC, BID	ulcers
Ciprofloxacin	20 – 40mg/kg PO, BID	antibiotic
Clavamox® (clavulinic acid/amoxicillin)	10-20 mg/kg (amoxi) PO, SID	antibiotic
Clindamycin	10mg/kg PO,BID	antibiotic
Clonazepam(Klonipin®)	1 mg/kg PO BID	fear, phobias
Comfortis®	1 tab PO monthly	flea control
Dexamethazone	.1 - .2 mg/kg SC,IV,IM, SID	steroid, anti-inflam.
Diazepam (Valium®)	1-2 mg/kg PO BID	anxiety,seizures
Diethylstilbesterol (DES)	1 mg PO x 3 days,then q 7 days	female incontinence
Diphenhydramine HCL	2 mg/kg q 4-12 hrs	allergy,anaphylaxis
Doxycycline	5 – 10 mg/kg SID	blood parasites,antibiotic
Enalapril	1 mg/kg SID (standard)	heart and kidney disease
Enrofloxacin (Baytril®)	5 – 10 mg/kg PO,SC,IM BID	antibiotic
Epinephrine(1/1000:1mg/ml)	.02 mg/kg SC (.01 ml/lb)	anaphylaxis, cardiac arrest
Famotidine (Pepsid®)	.5 – 1.0 mg/kg BID	ulcer
Fluoxetine(Prozac®)	1 mg/kg PO SID – BID	aggression, obsessive beh
Frontline®	topically q 3 – 4 weeks	fleas and ticks
Furosemide	2 mg/kg BID PO (6mg/kg IV once)	diuretic
Imidacloprid (Advantage®)	once topically q 3 – 4 weeks	flea control
Insulin (many kinds)	.5 – 1.0 mg/kg SC q 12 – 24 hrs	diabetes
Ivermectin	200µg/kg (.02 ml/kg) PO,SC SID ***Not for Collies, Shelties, Old English Sheepdogs***	mites, worms
Kaopectate	2 ml/kg PO q 4 – 6 hrs PRN	GI protectant
Ketoconazole	5 – 10 mg/kg SID or BID	antifungal
Lime Sulfur Dip	Mix as directed, dip q 7 days x 6	mange, other
Liquitinic®	1 ml/kg PO SID – BID	iron/vit. suppl.
Loperamide (Imodium®)	.1 - .2 mg/kg BID	antidiarrheal
Meloxicam (Metacam®)	.1 mg/kg SID	arthritis, analgesic
Metamucil® (Psyllium)	2 – 4 tbs/cup or can of food	bulk laxative
Methocarbamol (Robaxin®)	22 mg/kg PO TID	muscle relaxer
Metoclopramide	.2 - .5 mg/kg PO, SC TID	inc. gut motility antiemetic
Metronidazole	10 – 12 mg/kg PO BID	antiprotozoal
Maalox®	.5 ml/kg PO TID	antacid/ulcers
Miconazole	topically SID	antifungal
Mylanta®, Milk of Magnesia®	5 – 15 ml PO BID	antacid
Omeprazole (Prilosec®)	.5 - .7 mg/kg PO SID	ulcers

Orbifloxacin (Orbax®)	2.5 mg/kg PO SID	antibiotic
Pancreazyme®,Viokase®	Use as directed	enzyme supplement
Paroxetine(Paxil®)	1 mg/kg PO BID	antianxiety, compulsive disorder
Penicillin	20,000- 100,000 U/kg SQ,IM	antibiotic
Peptobismol® (bismuth subsalicylate)	.25 – 2.5 ml/kg PO TID	antidiarrheal
Praziquantel (Droncit®)	5 – 7.5 mg/kg PO once	tapeworms
Prednisone, prednisilone	usual dose .5 – 1.0 mg/kg	antiinflammatory
Promeris®	use as directed	fleas and ticks
Pyrantel Pamoate (Strongid T®,Nemex®)	5mg/kg PO. Repeat in 2 weeks	rounds, hookworms
Ranitidine (Zantac®)	2 – 5 mg/kg PO BID	ulcers
Selamectin(Revolution®)	topical q 30 days	HW prev.,fleas,ticks mange, int. worms
Selegiline (Anipryl®)	.5 mg/kg PO SID	cognitive dysfunction
Silver sulfadiazine (Silvadine®) Cream	topically SID or BID	burns
Sucralfate (Carafate®)	.5 – 1.0 grams PO BID	ulcers
Sulfadimethoxine(Albon®)	55 mg/kg PO SID x 10 days	coccidia
Sulfatrimethoprim	30 mg/kg PO SID	antibiotic
Tetracycline	10 – 25 mg/kg PO TID	antibiotic
Thyroxine (Synthroid®)	.02 mg/kg PO BID	hypothyroidism
Triamcinolone (Vetalog®)	.1-.2 mg/kg SC, IM once	antinflammatory
Vectra®	topically q 3 – 4 weeks	fleas and ticks
Vitamin B 12	200 μg PO SID	anemia
Vitamin E	400 – 1000 IU PO SID	antioxidant
Vitamin K1	2.5 mg/kg SID x 4 weeks	rat poison antidote

LEGEND

SID = once per day
BID = twice per day
TID = three times per day
Q = every (i.e. q 30days means every 30 days)
PO = by mouth
SC = subcutaneously
IM = intramuscularly
IV = intravenously
Mg = milligrams
Kg = kilograms
μg = micrograms
IU = international units

CALCULATING A DOSE: A KG = 2.2 POUNDS, SO DIVIDE A DOG'S WEIGHT IN POUNDS BY 2.2 THEN MULTIPLY BY THE DOSE LISTED. i.e. A 44 pound dog (44 ÷2.2) = 20kg, so if we see that the dose for metronidazole is 10 mg/kg, we would multiply 10 mg/kg by 20 kg to get a dose of 200 mg, and BID tells us that we would give it twice per day.

Grooming

Grooming dogs is often a very important part of their health maintenance protocol. The skin is the largest organ of a dog's body and matted hair may serve as the site for the beginning of a bad bacterial or fungal infection. Parasites such as ticks, fleas or lice may find a favorable environment in an unkempt fur coat, and certainly their reproduction is enhanced with prolonged survival on their unfortunate host. So bathe your dog as necessary with a shampoo recommended for dogs and have your pet groomed professionally on a regular basis. Admittedly, a long haired animal will require trimming more frequently than a short haired animal, but both will benefit from being kept clean and well groomed. **Fig 47**

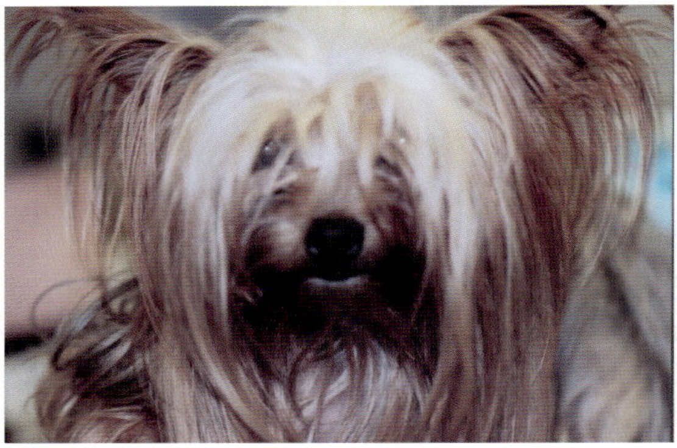

Fig. 47. Grooming. Many breeds require regular grooming in order to stay healthy.

Generally speaking, bathing should occur no more than once weekly unless the dog is receiving a medicated bath prescribed by a veterinarian. More frequent bathing will often result in the skin drying out, and this may lead to flaking and other problems.

Clipping will depend upon the dog and the groomer's recommendations. Grooming is as much of an art as a science, but most groomers have extensive training in performing trims that are both attractive and healthy for your dog.

Natural Medicine

There is a wealth of information available on natural or herbal cures for many of the problems discussed in this book. There is no doubt as to the effectiveness of optimal nutrition, including the use of organic foods in some cases, as well as herbal or homeopathic treatments in other cases. In addition, acupuncture and chiropractic techniques have been successfully utilized in many cases. However, this is beyond the scope of this book. I would encourage those who are interested in this approach to consult with a holistic veterinarian or herbal ist. I would also recommend a wonderful publication that summarizes many of these therapies: ***The Encyclopedia of Natural Pet Care by CJ Puotinen***.

Testing (What, When and Why Your Veterinarian will suggest tests)

Sometimes your veterinarian will suggest that certain tests be performed on your dog in order to help make a diagnosis and decide on a treatment plan. These tests may include a fecal exam, a skin scraping, bloodwork, a needle aspirate, a biopsy, a culture, a radiograph (X–ray), or a sonogram.
Fecal Exam: Checks for parasites and their eggs in the stool. This is a very important test to perform if vomiting or diarrhea is involved.

Skin Scraping: This test is literally just that; it is scraping the skin with a scalpel or other instrument to collect some of the material from the surface of the skin which will then be examined under the microscope. The main purpose of this test is to detect the presence of suspected mites on the skin, especially sarcoptic and demodectic mange mites.

Bloodwork: Several blood tests are commonly suggested in order to detect which organ is the source of the problems observed. A **CBC** (Complete Blood Count) is a way to rapidly scan all of the major cells circulating in the blood stream. Changes in the white blood cell numbers or types may suggest an infection is present, while a drop in the red cell numbers indicates anemia. Many other things may be determined from a CBC, including the presence of some cancers, exposure to certain poisons and allergic tendencies. A **Blood Chemistry (SMAC)** registers the level of different enzymes and other chemicals in the bloodstream and indicates metabolic or organ malfunctions. It essentially allows your veterinarian to "look inside" of your dog and see what isn't working or what is inflamed. When combined with a CBC, it is a very powerful diagnostic tool that can indicate where the trouble is and what it is likely to be! These tests may be recommended any time a dog is sick for any reason, especially if the signs are chronic in nature. A **Heartworm Test** is usually a test designed to pick up proteins produced by adult female heartworms present in the heart of your dog. These proteins are called antigens. This is a very sensitive kind of test that can identify the presence of worms even if there are no baby heartworms (microfilaria) in the blood. There are many other blood tests that your veterinarian may recommend but their discussion is beyond the scope of this book.

Needle Aspirate: A needle is inserted into a mass and the plunger is drawn back in an effort to remove cells which may then be placed on a slide and examined microscopically. Sometimes this can determine the presence and kind of tumor which may be present. This test is not invasive and may sometimes be performed without anesthesia. There are some drawbacks however, and sometimes the needle will miss the cells needed to make a diagnosis. In these cases a biopsy will be required.

Biopsy: A biopsy is the surgical removal of some tissue in order to examine it histologically. This allows for an accurate identification of the tissue in question and helps to determine what would be the best course of treatment.

Culture: In this case, a culture is when a swab is taken of an infected area in order to determine which organism is involved and which antibiotic may be the most effective in treating the problem. Cultures may look for bacteria or fungi, and there are a variety of different kinds of cultures. They are generally expensive, but well worth the expense.

Radiographs: Also known by the general public as X-rays, these are invaluable in diagnosing many problems. They allow a doctor to look inside your pet for tumors, foreign objects, heart and lung problems, fractures, dislocations and many other things.

Sonograms: Unlike a radiograph, a sonogram (ultrasound) gives a doctor a three dimensional view of the problem area. They are both more informative and more expensive.

Dog First Aid Kit

Activated Charcoal (liquid)
Baby scissors
Bandage scissors
Blanket
Tweezers
Rolled gauze bandage, gauze pads
Ace bandage/pet wrap
Syringes: 1cc, 3 cc, 5 cc, 20cc (good for medicating, feeding or flushing)
Styptic powder, soap, or corn starch, cyanoacrylate glue
Rectal thermometer
Vaseline
Nail clippers
Pedialyte®
Pepto Bismol®
Benadryl ®(diphenhydramine HCL) 25 mg caps or children's elixir
Saline eye wash
Stomach Tube
Towel and washcloth
Antibiotic ointment
Hydrocortisone ointment
Hydrogen peroxide
Rubbing alcohol
Ear mite medication
Muzzle
Extra Collar and leash
Penlight
Latex gloves
Ear syringe
Eye Dropper
Eye Rinse
Splint materials (wood, clean paint sticks,etc.)
Flea and tick topical agent
Dog Carrier

Chart of Normal Values (temperature, pulse and respiration which you have measured when your dog has been at rest in a non-emergency situation). Vet's phone number

Fast Dog Facts

Body Temperature	Adults: 101.5° F (textbook), range 100 -102.4 °F (37.7- 39.1°C) Puppies: Mid 90s ° F
Pulse (Heart Rate)	Large Dogs: 60 – 150 beats per minute Small Dogs: 70 – 180 BPM
Respiration	Large Dogs: 10 – 20 breaths per minute Small Dogs: 15 – 35 breaths per minute
Gut Transit Time	12 hours
Caloric Requirements	Puppies and young dogs: 180 – 260 kcals/kg Adults and older dogs: 60 kcals/kg *
Socialization Period	12 weeks (major windows to introduce children, cats, etc. Close at this age in many puppies).
Sexual Maturity	8 – 14 months
Estrus (Heat) frequency	5 – 10 months
Length of Estrus	2 – 20 days (usually around 10 days), proestrus lasts 2 – 11 days
Gestation	63 days
Termination of Estrus Cycles	7-9 years

*Dry foods usually supply about 1500 – 1700 kcal per pound of food, canned foods generally supply about 500 – 600 kcal per pound of food.

Some Helpful Dog Websites

www.aspca.org/apcc

www.akc.org

www.akcchf.org

www.doghobbyist.com

www.healthypet.com

www.avma.org

www.ofa.com

www.canismajor.com/dog

www.veterinarypartner.com

www.dog-first-aid-101.com

www.pets.ca/articles/aritcle-firstaidk9.htm (CPR guide and illustrations)

www.geocities.com/~olelo/shelties/emergencydoglinks.html
(Many useful links)

www.redcross-cmd.org/Chapter/petguiderev.html

www.veterinarypartner.com/content.plx?P=SRC&5=0&sourceID=6
(Good poison information)

www.prepare.org/animal/petaid.htm (Red Cross site with multiple languages)

www.peteducation.com/category.cfm?c-2+1677

Preventive Maintenance and Vaccination Protocol

Dogs, and especially puppies get into things. Puppy proof your house. That means that you should remove anything that might be eaten...that shouldn't be! This includes foam matting, soft rubber objects, small chewable objects, electric cords within reach, insect or rodent poisons, medicines and bottles of cleaning agents. Plastic bags, sheets, or anything else made of plastic are all likely to be irresistible to puppies. Physical threats include objects that fall over, doors that close automatically and falls. Swimming pools and hot tubs also represent a threat for small dogs that may not be able to get out easily if they fall in.

Escaping leads to a whole series of potential risks that include everything from being hit by a car to getting into fights with other dogs, cats, or wild animals. Vaccinations are important, especially for distemper and parvo, but most veterinarians will vaccinate for these as well as infectious canine hepatitis, leptospirosis, coronavirus, infectious tracheobronchits (kennel cough) and rabies. Other vaccinations may be recommended depending upon your dogs risk factors and geographic location i.e. Lyme Disease is much more common in the Northeastern United States than it is in the southern parts of the country. Without vaccinations, these viral diseases may be fatal. Even if not fatal, treatment may be very expensive and sometimes permanent damage may occur even if the dog survives. Initial vaccinations usually start around 6 weeks of age and often involves vaccinations every 2 weeks until 3 – 4 months of age. Annual vaccinations are recommended after that.

Kennel Cough (*Bordetella*) vaccinations may be recommended every 6 months in some areas.

Older dogs, or those that reside indoors (particularly those in urban areas), may not require vaccinations annually. However, since the incidence of infectious diseases varies from place to place, consult with your veterinarian.

Recently, rabies vaccines have been developed that provide protection for three years. Therefore many counties have dropped the requirement for annual rabies vaccinations and instead require vaccinations only every three years. Consult with your veterinarian however, in case you live in a high incidence rabies area.

Parasite control is essential in order to maintain good health. Some veterinarians recommend an initial deworming at 2 weeks of age, and then again at 4 weeks of age. Certainly, puppies are very likely to get worms from their mothers before they are even eating solid food, so this approach makes sense. As far as external parasites are concerned, there are a number of very effective flea control products available. Some of these also help to control ticks. These are discussed in more detail in the section on fleas and ticks. Use them regularly and check your dog regularly to make sure that they are working.

Heartworms are deadly or at the very least debilitating. Get your dog on heartworm prevention early and give it regularly. Have your dog checked for these worms every year during the annual check up.

Speaking of annual checkups, these are very important. The sooner a problem is identified, the easier it will be to repair. For older dogs, an annual geriatric blood screen is extremely helpful in discovering problems before they become too serious. I strongly recommend geriatric blood screening and also recommend regular bloodwork for any dog that is on regular medication. Indeed, this is also advised by the American Animal Hospital Association.

Dental disease is a common and serious problem in dogs. If left untreated it can result in tooth loss, mouth infection, bone infection or a heart infection. Regular dental cleaning are advisable but the frequency of the cleanings will depend upon the individual dog. Preventing periodontal disease in this manner will help to protect the heart, liver and kidneys from damage, and may extend the lifespan of the dog considerably.

Prevent overheating. **Do not leave a dog in a parked car with the windows closed or even cracked open for any more than 5 minutes!** Even 5 minutes may be too much time in some circumstances. If you must leave your dog in the car for more than 5 minutes, leave the air conditioner on, and keep the windows open just a bit. This is only a problem during the daytime.

Occasionally, allergic reactions occur to vaccinations. While this is fairly rare, it is often manifested by swelling of the face and hives on the rest of the body. It may also be accompanied by vomiting and diarrhea. In severe cases, anaphylactic shock may occur. This is recognized by pale gums, and generalized weakness. *See the section on Treating Insect Bites for the treatment of anaphylactic shock*. First aid generally involves the use of Benadryl®, steroids, and epinephrine--the doses are listed in the Drug Chart.

Veterinary Poisoning Advice Numbers

ASPCA National Animal Poison Control Center 1 (800) 548-2423

Pet Poison Helpline 1 (800) 213-6680

References

Anonymous. First Aid for Our Best Friends. 2001. Doris Day Animal League. Washington, D.C. 95 pp.

ASPCA. 2009. 101 Things You Didn't Know Could Harm Your Pet. ASPCA Pet Health Insurance Pamphlet. 14 pp.

Boothe, Dawn. 2000. Boothe's Small Animal Formulary. 5th Edition. AAHA Press. Lakewood, CO 244 pp.

Campbell, A. and M. Chapman. 2000. Handbook of Poisoning in Dogs and Cats. Blackwell Science. 272 pp.

Eldredge, D.M., L. Carlson, D. Carlson and J. Giffin. 2007. Dog Owner's Home Veterinary Handbook. Fourth Edition. Wiley Publishing Co. Hoboken, New Jersey. 628 pp.

Ettinger, Stephen J. 1993. Pocket Companion to Textbook of Veterinary Internal Medicine. W.B. Saunders. Philadelphia. 892 pp.

Fenner, William R. 1982. Quick Reference to Veterinary Medicine. Lippincott Company. Philadelphia. 592 pp.

Goldston, Richard and Johnny Hoskins. 1995. Geriatrics and Gerontology of the Dog and Cat. W.B. Saunders. Philadelphia. 426 pp.

Hanel, Rita. 2008. Common questions in cardiopulmonary cerebral resuscitation. Clinician's Brief. NAVC. October, 2008(6)10:21-22.

Johnson, Norman H. and Saul Galin. 1977. The Complete Puppy and Dog Book. Atheneum. New York. 490 pp.

Keuhn, Ned F.(Ed.). 2004. North American Companion Animal Formulary. Sixth Edition. North American Compendiums, Inc. Port Huron, Mich. 248 pp.

Kirk, Robert and Stephen Bistner. 1985. Veterinary Procedures and Emergency Treatment. W.B. Saunders. Philadelphia. 1000 pp.

Lewis, Lon and Mark Morris. 1984. Small Animal Clinical Nutrition. Mark Morris Associates. Topeka, Kansas.

Melman, Stephen. 1994. Skin Diseases of Dogs and Cats. Dermapet Inc. Potomac, Maryland. 264 pp.

Preston, Gilbert. 1997. Wilderness First Aid. Falcon Globe Pequot Press. Guilford, Connecticut. 126 pp.

Puotinen, CJ. 1997. The Encyclopedia of Natural Pet Care. Keats Publishing Inc. New Canaan, Connecticut. 522 PP.

INDEX

Notes